I0450193

Autoimmune Disease Anti-Inflammatory Diet

Chronic Pain Relief

3rd Edition

By Mary Solomon

© **Copyright 2014- Mary Solomon - All rights reserved.**

In no way is it legal to reproduce, duplicate, or transmit any part of this document in either electronic means or in printed format. Recording of this publication is strictly prohibited and any storage of this document is not allowed unless with written permission from the publisher. All rights reserved.

The information provided herein is stated to be truthful and consistent, in that any liability, in terms of inattention or otherwise, by any usage or abuse of any policies, processes, or directions contained within is the solitary and utter responsibility of the recipient reader. Under no circumstances will any legal responsibility or blame be held against the publisher for any reparation, damages, or monetary loss due to the information herein, either directly or indirectly.

Respective authors own all copyrights not held by the publisher.

Legal Notice:

This eBook is copyright protected. This is only for personal use. You cannot amend, distribute, sell, use, quote or paraphrase any part or the content within this eBook without the consent of the author or copyright owner. Legal action will be pursued if this is breached.

Disclaimer Notice:

Please note the information contained within this document is for educational and entertainment purposes only. Every attempt has been made to provide accurate, up to date and reliable complete information. No warranties of any kind are expressed or implied. Readers acknowledge that the author is not engaging in the rendering of legal, financial or professional advice.

By reading this document, the reader agrees that under no circumstances are we responsible for any losses, direct or indirect, which are incurred as a result of the use of information contained within this document, including, but not limited to, —errors, omissions, or inaccuracies.

Contents

Introduction

Chapter 1: What Are Autoimmune Diseases?

Chapter 2: What is an AutoImmune Disease and Can I Survive One

Chapter 3: General Characteristics

Chapter 4: Do You Have An Autoimmune Disease?

Chapter 5: Cancer As Autoimmune Disorder

Chapter 6: All About Inflammation

Chapter 7: Major Components of Inflammation

Chapter 8: Events That Occur After Acute Inflammation

Chapter 9: Process Of Chronic Inflammation

Chapter 10: Inflammation and Pain

Chapter 11: Possible Treatments for Inflammation

Chapter 12: What is an Anti-Inflammatory Diet?

Chapter 13: Eating On The Anti-Inflammatory Diet

Chapter 14: Where To Find Recipes?

PART 2 - Gluten

Chapter 15: Gluten Sensitivity vs. Celiac Disease

Chapter 16: Living Gluten-Free

Chapter 17: How to Get Started on a Gluten-Free Diet

Chapter 18 - Quick Start Guide - What You Can and Can't Eat

Chapter 19: How to Manage Your Gluten-Free Lifestyle

Chapter 20: Supplements for a Gluten-Free Dieter

Conclusion

Appendix

References

Introduction

Thank you and congratulations for purchasing the Autoimmune Disease and Anti-inflammatory Diet Book. If you are like me and the millions of other people suffering from an autoimmune disease, you are desperate to find relief from multiple symptoms. After twenty-five years of suffering from symptoms like severe exhaustion, arthritis and joint pain, body aches, nausea, headaches, weight loss, brain fog, and neuropathy, I discovered a diet that has relieved of all of these symptoms. Yes, every single one of them! And it can work for you, too!

Over the last several years, modern medicine is just now discovering that what we eat can often by the catalyst or culprit to our autoimmune diseases. The very foods we've been told were good for us are making many of us sick. The FDA cannot decide whether or not specific foods cause issues and their opinion changes continuously about the various symptoms associated with ingesting various foods when you have an underlying illness.

I would notice that my symptoms increased when I at certain foods. "How could that be?" I asked. My family and friends eat these items and they aren't sick. It was difficult for me to believe that something as simple as changing my diet could change my life and possibly extend my life by decades, while increasing my comfort level.

I encourage you to give it a chance! It can work for you, too; whether you have lupus, multiple sclerosis, Sjogren's syndrome, rheumatoid arthritis, or any of the many other autoimmune disorders. This diet can work for you and I know you will experience a change almost instantly when you drop the foods that are causing you more difficulty than your disease is.

Now, let's understand what inflammation is!

The word inflammation is derived from the Latin word, 'inflammo', which means 'I set alight, I ignite'. It is one of the complex biological responses of vascular tissues to the various harmful stimuli like pathogens, damaged cells or irritants. It is the response of body's immune system against internal or external stimulus.

Inflammation is a protective response of the body involving mediators, blood vessels, host cells and proteins, and it is an attempt of the body to remove initial causes of the cell injury, necrotic cells and the damaged tissues because of initial injury, and to start the healing process.

When any harmful or irritating substance attacks any part of our body, the body's immune system is activated that tries to remove that harmful substance. The signs of inflammation we see initially, more specifically when it comes to acute inflammation, are the indications that our body is trying to heal own its own.

Without inflammation, our body cannot heal, but when it becomes out of control, as in autoimmune diseases like rheumatoid arthritis, it can damage the body. Basically, with an autoimmune disease, your body sees itself as a threat and begins attacking itself. This is the most damaging form of inflammation because it becomes a non-stop fight of your immune system verses your own body systems and your joints.

Change your diet in order to change your life! You're worth it and you deserve to feel better! While there are over 80 different types of autoimmune disorders noted in medical text, we will only be covering a certain number of them in-depth in this book. We will however list the individual disorders as a whole to give you an idea of how many different disorders are actually known of today and how many that modern medicine can successfully treat and create comfort for. You will be amazed at how many actually plague the population, and how many medical science has identified over the last several years.

Chapter 1: What Are Autoimmune Diseases?

Whether you're curious about autoimmune diseases or you want to find a way to heal a current autoimmune disease, you're in the right place! An autoimmune disease develops when our immune system attacks healthy body cells and causes severe damage to the muscles, nerves and tissue in the affected area.

Normally, our immune system is a defense against harmful germs, bacteria, viruses, etc., and its job is to make sure our body is protected from foreign invaders. Bearing that in mind, when an autoimmune disease develops, our immune system does the opposite of what it was biologically programmed to do. Instead of attacking foreign cells, it begins attacking healthy cells, leaving the body at risk for infection from outside sources, since the immune system is already preoccupied.

Types of Autoimmune Diseases

Currently, approximately 80 known autoimmune diseases have been discovered but researchers are certain that there are more going undiscovered everyday. While there are quite a few known autoimmune diseases, there are some that are more common than others. A few common ones are:

- Sjogren's syndrome - Attacks moisture producing glands. Can also attack other areas such as the lungs, kidneys, and neurological system;
- Multiple sclerosis – The protective coating around the nerves along the spinal cord are damaged by the immune system;
- Psoriasis – This is a disease that affects the skin. Causes an over production of skin cells creating red, itchy, painful patches over the entire body. Can also cause arthritis;
- Rheumatoid arthritis – Immune system attacks the joints. Can also attack the lungs, kidneys and blood vessels.
- Lupus - Can attack many parts to the body, including skin, joints, blood vessels and kidneys.
- Scleroderma – This disease causes the blood vessels and connective tissue to grow abnormally, causing trouble swallowing, shortness of breath, skin abnormalities, etc;
- Inflammatory Bowel Disease (IBD) – Includes Crohn's disease and ulcerative colitis. Can cause abdominal pain, vomiting, bloating, diarrhea, rectal bleeding, etc;
- Hashimoto's disease – This disease affects the thyroid causing the thyroid gland to under produce thyroid hormone.

- Transplant Rejection: Almost all sorts of transplant operations cause inflammation. If the immune system of the person receiving the organ rejects the donated organ, the inflammation occurs in the transplanted organ and in the surrounding tissues.
- Various Allergic Reactions: All allergic reactions cause inflammation. Asthma causes inflammation of the airways, hay fever causes inflammation in nose, ear, throat and mucous membranes. People that are sensitive or allergic to bee stings must avoid bees because if they get a bee sting, it can develop a serious life threatening allergic response known as anaphylactic shock.
- Type 1 Diabetes: If diabetes is left unchecked and not managed appropriately, inflammation in various parts of the body can develop quickly.
- Celiac Disease: This immune disease involves destruction and inflammation in the inner lining of the small intestine.

Let us look at these and some more conditions under the autoimmune disease category, as well as how they have an effect on our body in detail.

Sjogren's Disease

Sjogren's disease is another disease that is considered to be an autoimmune disease. This is a disorder of the immune system and it is identified by the two of its most common symptoms that include dry mouth and dry eyes. This syndrome is one that will often happen with other disorders of the immune system including lupus and rheumatoid arthritis. Typically it is referred to as a comorbid disease or a secondary disorder. In this syndrome, the moisture secreting glands that are present in the eyes and the mouth as well as the mucous membranes are the parts that are affected first which will result in a decreased production of the saliva and tears in the sufferer.

While it is possible to develop Sjogren's syndrome at any age, the majority of sufferers will be those who are older than 40 years of age at the time they are diagnosed because this is the time that symptoms generally present. The condition is also more commonly found in women than men and it has also been proven that men present symptoms of the disease later than women. The treatment that is usually given will focus on relieving the symptoms that the affected person has.

The two main symptoms that were reported with this disorder include dry eyes and dry mouth. For those who have issues with the dry eyes, it is common to feel that your eyes are burning, feeling gritty, and itching. You might feel like there is sand in your eyes. For those who are having issues with their dry mouth, you are going to feel like your mouth is full of cotton that can make it really difficult to speak or to swallow.

There are a few other symptoms that you might experience with this syndrome including prolonged fatigue, persistent dry cough, vaginal dryness, skin rashes and dry skin, salivary glands that are swollen, especially the set that are right behind your jaw and in front of your ears. Other common symptoms are joint stiffness, swelling, and pain.

For those who are dealing with disorder, it means that the immune system is attacking the tissues and the cells that are inside your body. There is no clear research that is able to prove why some people are going to develop Sjogren's syndrome while others are not. There are some genes that will put people at a higher risk of getting this disorder, but it seems that this is not enough to cause it at all times; many people will have the necessary gene but will not have the disorder. Which can sometimes cause the test for the disorder to show up as a false positive, causing the true disorder to go undiagnosed for months, or possibly years. It is thought by most diagnosticians that the gene has to be coupled with some triggering mechanism, such as a bacteria or virus, in order to activate the disorder in the immune system or for symptoms to begin to develop. This is why it is thought that some people with the gene develop the disorder, while others do not.

With Sjogren's syndrome, your immune system is going to start by first targeting the glands that secrete the moisture in your mouth and in your eyes. But it is then going to start attacking other parts of your body. These other parts might include the nerves, skin, lungs, liver, kidneys, thyroid, and joints. Although it is possible for anyone to develop this syndrome, it is more likely to occur in those who have at least one of the known risk factors, if not more. These risk factors would include things such as:

- Age—those who develop this syndrome are usually those who are above the age of 40.
- Sex—it is much more common to find this disorder in women compared to men.
- Rheumatic disease—it is very common for those who are suffering from this disease to also have issues with other rheumatic disease such as lupus or arthritis.

Those who have a combination of these three factors are much more likely to get this disorder at some point in their lives. It is important to talk to your doctor about your risk factors and start to follow the diet requirements that are listed later in this guidebook. The earlier that you begin the diet that is outlined in this book, the less likely you will be to see extreme symptoms. Starting this diet early will also help you to see the best results.

Multiple Sclerosis

Multiple Sclerosis is another disease that can be caused by the immune system attacking your body. In the case of this disorder, the immune system is going to be attacking the myelin, or the protective sheath, that covers up your nerves. This myelin damage is going to cause a disruption in the communication between the brain and the rest of the body. Over time, the nerves are going to start deteriorating, a process that is not reversible with modern medicine.

The signs and symptoms that the sufferer may be dealing with will vary by quite a bit and will often depend on the amount of the damage and which of the nerves have been affected. Some people who are further progressed with this disorder may not have the ability to walk independently and others may go through long periods where they are in remission and they are not developing any new symptoms at all.

As of right now, there are no cures that are available for multiple sclerosis. However, there are treatments that can help speed up the time that it takes to recover from attacks, can help to modify the course of the disease, and to help manage symptoms.

The symptoms and signs of this disorder are going to vary, often depending on the location of the nerve fibers that have been affected. Some of the symptoms that might be discovered would include:

- Weakness or numbness in one or more of the limbs. This is usually going to occur on one side of the body at a time.
- Either a complete or a partial loss of vision and it will usually occur just in one eye and the progress over to the other one later. Many sufferers will complain that this is also coupled with pain when moving the eye.
- Blurring of the vision or double vision.
- Tingling or some pain in various parts of the body that will not go away.
- Sensations that feel like electric-shock that are going to occur when certain neck movements are attempted. This usually happens when the neck is being bent forward.
- A tremor or a lack of coordination. It can also include an unsteady gait
- Problems with bladder or bowel function
- Dizziness
- Fatigue
- Slurred speech

Most of the people who are dealing with this disorder will have a relapsing and remitting disease course. Any new symptoms, or the relapse, can develop over days or even weeks and over time they might improve completely or partially. Once the relapse has improved a bit, there is usually going to be a quiet period, or the remission, that will last for a variation of time, sometimes for a few months and sometimes even longer. At times, small increases in the temperature of the body might cause a worsening of the symptoms, but this is not considered a relapse.

Around 60 percent of those who are in a relapsing and remitting cycle will at some point develop a progression of symptoms that is more progressive; these may or may not include periods of remission. These worsening symptoms will usually include some issues with gait and the rate of this progression is going to vary quite a bit among people who are dealing with this secondary progressive form of the disorder.

There are some people with this disorder who will experience a slow onset as well as a steady progression of the signs and symptoms of MS without any relapse. This is known as primary progressive MS. Each of the sufferers are going to go through the process in a different way.

Some will feel certain symptoms that others will not. Some will take years to get really bad and others will go through the progression really quickly. The areas of the body that are affected, as well as how advanced the attack is from the immune system is going to affect how the person handles the disorder as well as how quickly they will go downhill.

The causes of this disorder are still unknown. It is known that this is an autoimmune disease where the body can start to attack the tissues that are inside. It is also unclear why some people will develop this disorder while others will not. There are some guesses as to what this can be, such as childhood infections or genetics, but it is still clinically undetermined.

If someone you know develops this disorder, it is a good idea to seek help right away. While there is no known cure for this disorder, it is possible to get help in order to slow down the progression and to alleviate any of the symptoms that the sufferer might be going through. It is also a good idea for the family to get the help that they need in dealing with this situation as it worsens.

Psoriasis

Psoriasis is another autoimmune disorder, although it does not cause the same kind of life altering issues that are found in multiple sclerosis. Psoriasis is a common condition of the skin that is going to change the life cycle of these skin cells. This disorder is one that is going to cause the cells to build up very quickly on the surface of the skin. These extra skin cells are going to form into silvery and thick scales as well as red, dry, and itchy patches that can sometimes cause pain to the sufferer.

Psoriasis is a disease that is going to be persistent and long lasting. In some patients there are times when you will be able to get relief from the symptoms of this disorder, but that is going to alternate with times when the symptoms are getting worse. There is no cure for this disorder, but there are a few treatments that work in order to stop the skin from growing as quickly and can offer quite a bit of relief to the patient.

Lifestyle measures can also be taken into account in order to help; these would include using cortisone creams and making sure to expose your skin to a little bit of natural sunlight. These actions can help with the symptoms of psoriasis.

The signs and symptoms that can come from psoriasis are going to vary between the people who are dealing with this disease. Some of the things that you should watch out for include:

- Stiff and swollen joints
- Ridged, pitted, and thickened nails
- Soreness, burning, or itching
- Dry and cracked skin that might be prone to bleeding
- Small spots of scales (this is usually seen in children)
- Red patches that are all over the skin and that are covered with silvery scales.

There are several different types of psoriasis that you may come across. These are going to be discussed in further detail below.

Plaque Psoriasis
This is the form that is the most common. It is going to cause red, raised, and dry skin legions or plaques that are covered with silvery scales. The plaque is often going to itch or it can get really painful and you will be able to find it on any area of our body; this would include areas such as the soft tissues that are in your mouth and your genitals. It is also possible to have one small spot of this psoriasis or many of them all over the body.

Nail Psoriasis
Psoriasis is not something that is just going to affect the direct skin of your body; it can also take effect on your toenails and fingernails. When it does, it is going to cause discoloration, abnormal growth of the nail, and pitting. Psoriasis of the nail may, at times, cause the nail to become loose and then separate out from the nail bed. In some of the most severe cases, this disorder can cause the nail to completely crumble.

Scalp Psoriasis

If you are dealing with psoriasis of the scalp, you are going to have a scalp that appears and looks itchy and red and then is topped with some silvery white scales. The scaly and red areas are often going to extend further than the hairline so it can be noticed on your face or on your neck. You may also notice that there are flakes of dead skin throughout your hair or on your shoulders, especially once you are done scratching the top of your head.

Psoriatic arthritis

This is another stage of the disorder that is going to cause some more pain and discomfort in the person who is affected. In addition to dealing with the scaly and inflamed skin, those who have psoriatic arthritis are also going to have to deal with painful and swollen joints, as well as discolored and pitted nails like others who are dealing with arthritis. Symptoms of this autoimmune disorder will often range from either mild or severe and this form of arthritis is able to affect any of the joints. Although this specific type of arthritis is not usually as crippling as some of the other types of arthritis, it is still able to cause progressive joint damage and stiffness in the sufferer and in some of the most severe cases it can lead to a permanent deformity of some sort, typically around the joints.

If you are dealing with psoriasis, you may be confused about when you should go and visit a doctor. Some good suggestions include:

- If you start to suspect that you are dealing with this disorder, you should go in and visit your doctor in

11

order to have an examination. If you already have this disorder, you should talk to them about it.

- If the psoriasis begins to progress beyond just being a nuisance. IF you are starting to feel some discomfort or pain with the disorder, you should seek help right away.
- If it is becoming difficult to perform some regular tasks throughout the day.
- If you are concerned about the way that your skin is appearing.
- If the start to have issues with your joints due to the disorder. This could include things like the inability to perform your daily tasks, swelling, and pain.

If any of the symptoms and signs that you have due to this disorder seem to be getting worse or any of the treatments are not working well for you, it is a good idea to get some medical advice as soon as possible. If you feel that your medication or combination of treatments is not working to help with the psoriasis, it is a good idea to talk with your doctor to discuss some other options that are available for you.

Rheumatoid arthritis

The next type of autoimmune disease that can be an issue is known as rheumatoid arthritis. This is an inflammatory disorder that is chronic and that is going to usually affect the small joints that are present in your feet and hands. Unlike the wear and tear damage that occurs with osteoarthritis, this kind of arthritis is going to affect the lining that is in the joints that can cause a painful swelling that will eventually result in erosion of the bone and deformity of the joint.

This disorder is one that occurs when the immune system starts to attack the tissues in your own body. In addition to being difficult on your joints, this disorder may at times affect other parts and organs of your body. These parts can include the blood vessels, lungs, eyes, and skin. Although this disorder is able to occur at any age in your life, it is more common to happen after the age of 40. The disorder is another one that is more common in women than in men.

The treatment that is given for this disorder is focused on preventing joint damage and controlling the symptoms so that the sufferer is not dealing with as much pain. Some of the symptoms and signs that you may experience with this disorder include:

- Swollen, warm, and tender joints.
- Stiffness that occurs in the morning but which is going to last for many hours
- Weight loss, fever, and fatigue
- Firm bumps that form in the tissue that is under the skin on your arms or the joints of your feet.

The early form of this disease is going to start out by affecting the smaller joints first, such as the ones that attach the toes to the feet and the fingers to the hands. As the disease continues to progress, the symptoms are going to spread to other parts of the body such as the shoulders, hips, elbows, ankles, knees, and wrists.

In most of these cases, the symptoms are going to occur in the same joints on each side of the body. The signs and symptoms that come from this disorder are going to vary in the severity that the person feels and in some cases it may come and go. Periods of increased activity of the disorder, also known as flares, will often alternate with periods of remission where the pain and the swelling are going to disappear. Over some time, the disorder may cause the joints to shift out of place and deform.

It is a good idea to visit your doctor as soon as possible if you are feeling persistent swelling and discomfort in your joints. There are medicines that are available that can help you to not feel as much pain and to slow down the progression of this disease so that it is more manageable.

Inflammatory Bowel Disease

Inflammatory bowel disease is when there is chronic inflammation in at least part if not all of the digestive tract. This disorder is going to mostly be classified as Crohn's disease or ulcerative colitis. Both of these are going to involve severe weight loss, fatigue, pain, and diarrhea. Depending on how this disorder is progressing, it can become debilitating and will sometimes lead to complications that can be life threatening.

Ulcerative colitis is one of the variations of this disease that causes inflammation that is long lasting, as well as sores or ulcers in the inner most lining of the colon or large intestine and rectum. Another form of IBD is Crohn's disease that is a form of this disorder that is going to cause inflammation in the lining of the digestive tract.

In this disease, the inflammation is going to spread deep into the tissue that is affected. The inflammation can sometimes involve various different areas in the digestive tract such as in the small intestine, large intestine or even both.

There are a lot of different signs and symptoms that can be indicative to having this disorder. These would include:

- Diarrhea—this is one of the most common symptoms that people with this disorder are going to be dealing with.
- Fatigue and fever—many of the sufferers of this disorder intermittently run a low grade to mid-grade fever. At times this can also lead to low energy levels which are going to make you feel very tired.
- Cramping and abdominal pain—ulceration and inflammation in your intestines is able to affect the normal movements of various contents through the digestive tract. When you are not able to get these normal movements, you may start to feel cramping and pain. They can also lead to vomiting and nausea in some cases.
- Blood in stools—at times you may notice that there is bright red blood that goes into the toilet or a darker blood that is mixed in with the stool. There are times when you will be bleeding and not notice it. It is good to seek medical help if this occurs to you.
- Reduced appetite—when you are going through the cramping and the abdominal pain as well as all of the inflammation, it is going to affect the appetite that you have.
- Unintentional weight loss—it is possible to lose a lot of weight and perhaps become extremely malnourished over a long term basis when you have this disorder. This is because you are not able to properly digest and then absorb the food that you are taking in due to this disorder.

As was mentioned a little bit above, there are a few different types of this disorder that you might be going through. Even with all of the different kinds of inflammatory bowel disease, they are all caused by the same thing; they are due to the fact that the immune system is working against your body by attacking it. Most of the treatments that are out there are meant to help make the symptoms easier to deal with and slow down the progression of the disorder. Here are some of the most common types of this disorder that you might come across.

Ulcerative Colitis
The first type of this disorder is known as ulcerative colitis. This is classified by the location of the inflammation as well as the severity of the symptoms that the sufferer is dealing with.

The specific symptoms one would experience from ulcerative colitis are:

- Loss of bowel movements, with our without blood
- Urgency of bowel movements and possible bowel incontinence
- Discomfort in the lower stomach, possible cramps
- Low grade fever, lethargy and loss of apetite
- Diarrhea accompanied by weight loss
- Anemia caused by bowel movements containing blood

Once the disorder begins attacking the immune system, other symptoms may develop, such as:

- Problems with vision
- Pain in the eyes

- Variety of joint disorders
- Neck pain
- Lower back pain
- Rash anywhere on the skin
- Liver disease
- Bile duct disease
- Kidney problems
- Blood or mucus in the stool
- Severe abdominal or rectal pain
- Dehydration
- Frequent bowel movements that are loose
- Progressively looser bowel movements

Ulcerative Proctitis

This is a type of the disorder where the inflammation that is felt is going to be confined to the area that is right next to the anus or the rectum. This is form, there may be some rectal bleeding and it is often the only sign that this disorder is going on. This form of the disorder is usually going to be the mildest.

Symptoms of Ulcerative Proctitis are:
- Diarrhea
- Bleeding
- The urge to empty the bowels, even when there is no stool present
- Mucus discharge
- Pain in the rectum
- Accidental Leakage from the Bowel

Proctosigmoiditis

This is a type of the disorder that is going to involved inflammation in the sigmoid colon, or the lower end of the colon, and the rectum. Symptoms and signs of this type of the disorder are going to include abdominal cramping, diarrhea, and issues with moving the bowels even though you feel that there is an urge to do this.

Symptoms of Proctosigmoiditis are:
- Inflammation in the rectum
- Inflammation in the sigmoid colon
- Rectal bleeding
- Urgency in bowel movements
- Bloody diarrhea with cramps

Left sided Colitis

This is a type of the disorder where the inflammation is going to extend from the rectum and then go up through the sigmoid as well as the descending colon. There are various symptoms and signs that can be found in this form of the disorder and they might include weight loss that is not intentional, pain on the left side of the body, abdominal cramping, and bloody diarrhea.

Symptoms of Left Sided Colitis include:
- Inflammation in the rectum, spreading up the left colon, into the sigmoid colon and descending colon.
- Bloody diarrhea
- Abdominal cramps
- Unintentional weight loss
- Left sided abdominal pain

Pancolitis

Pancolitis, also known as universal colitis affects the entire colon. This is the type of the disease that is going to affect the whole of the colon. There are some severe symptoms that can come with this disorder which includes significant weight loss due to the fact that you are not able to absorb and digest the food that you are consuming, fatigue, pain and abdominal cramps, and bloody diarrhea that can be really severe.

Other symptoms of pancolitis are:
- Bloody diarrhea
- Abdominal pain
- Cramps
- Unintentional weight loss
- Fatigue
- Fever
- Night sweats

Fulminant Colitis
This is a rare form of pancolitis. Most patients who have fulminant colitis become extremely ill. Patients suffer through extreme symptoms that range from mild to extremely severe or fatal.

Symptoms of Fulminant Colitis include:
- Dehydration
- Severe abdominal pain
- Protracted diarrhea with blood
- Possible shock
- Development of toxic megacolon
- Colonic rupture

Many patients are frequently hospitalized and given intervenous medications. Typically, when the symptoms of the disease become severe, the most affected pieces of the bowel are removed surgically to prevent rupture.

Acute Severe Ulcerative Colitis

This is a type of the disease that is going to affect the whole of the colon. It used to be known as fulminant colitis. The symptoms that come with this disorder are really severe. These will include the inability to eat, fever, bleeding, profuse diarrhea, and severe pain.

Other symptoms of Acute Severe Ulcerative Colitis are:
- Diarrhea, containing blood or pus
- Abdominal pain
- Cramping
- Pain in the rectum
- Bleeding from the rectum
- Urgency to use the restroom
- Inability to defecate
- Unintentional weight loss
- Fatigue
- Fever
- Failure to grow (in children)

Crohn's Disease

This is the final type of this disorder that can cause a lot of havoc on your body. This disease is going to involve inflammation in various parts of the digestive tract and each person is going to have it occur in a different part of the digestive tract. The parts that are the most commonly affected are the colon and the last little part found in the small intestine.

The inflammation can sometimes be confined to the bowel wall, which is going to lead to the narrowing to occur due to scarring, inflammation, or from both at the same time. At times, this may even swell through the bowel walls. The narrowing can at times lead to a blockage that can cause a lot of issues and pain. It is best to seek help as soon as possible for this.

Even with modern science, the cause of most autoimmune diseases is still unknown. However, a few theories include bacteria, drugs, and environmental elements. Although there are numerous autoimmune diseases, they all have one thing in common: they target and harm certain parts of the body, causing the body to deteriorate. There are medications to help ease the symptoms from these autoimmune diseases, but that's not the only way to help yourself. A simple diet change can improve your life forever.

If you are dealing with any of these conditions, it is important to keep in contact with your doctor in order to get the right treatment. It is also a good idea to see your doctor if you are dealing with a persistent change in the way your bowels work or if you have any of the symptoms or the signs that were described above for this disorder. Although this kind of disorder is not usually fatal, it is a disease that is serious and in some of the cases it can cause complications that are life threatening. Go in and get assistance right away so that you are able to get the symptoms in check before the issues become even more difficult to deal with.

These are just a few of the autoimmune diseases that you may come across. All of them are going to cause a lot of pain and issues with the body due to the fact that the immune system has for some reason decided that it is going to attack the different parts of your body. The reasons that cause most of these disorders are unknown; anyone is able to get them and have to deal with the symptoms at any time. There might be a couple of things that make you more likely to develop any of these disorders, such as being over the age of 40 and a woman, it is still unsure why some people will develop this disorder while others are not going to.

In addition, there are no known cures to these disorders and for the most part the treatments that are currently available are meant to help slow down the progress of the disease or to help you to not feel as much pain as it goes through its progression. Each person is going to experience these disorders in a different way. Some are going to go through the progression really quickly while others might have flare ups that come and go away and still others are going to experience them for years without them going away.

One of the safest ways that you will be able to deal with these kinds of disorders without having to take a lot of harmful medicine is to alter the types of foods that you eat and avoid foods that are known to cause inflammation. Earlier in this guidebook there was talk about the gluten free diet, which is a good diet plan that you can try out if you are dealing with some of these types of disorders. There is also an anti-inflammatory diet that you can try out that is helpful in reducing the times that you have pain and flair ups from your condition. The important thing that you are going to need to remember when you go on these diets is that they are more like habit changes than a regular diet.

You are not going to be able to go off them without having to deal with all of the pain and inflammation that you were supposed to be avoiding in the process. The diet that is discussed in the next few chapters talk about what you need to do such as limiting or completely getting rid of any of the foods that might cause inflammation in the body

Before getting started on this diet plan to help with your inflammation, or any other diet, you should take time to talk to your doctor. You do not want to get started on something that could end up causing more harm than good and your doctor is going to want to make sure that you are doing the diet in the right way and monitoring you the whole way.

Chapter 2: What is an AutoImmune Disease and Can I Survive One

There is a great deal of this book written with the basic understanding that you know what an autoimmune disease is, or as though you have done research into the disorders and understand the basics of how the immune system works. However, I think this is the perfect opportunity to take time out and break things down into laymans terms in an effort to help you develop a better understanding of what an automimmune disease really is and how you can survive life while suffering with one.

Being diagnosed with an autoimmune disease does not mean that you are being sentenced to a life of misery. There are many different treatments available to help manage autoimmune diseases and help create comfort while you are going through the ups and downs, or flares of the disease. It is important that you do not give into the rumors that everyone with an autoimmune disease suffers greatly. If caught early enough, treatment is extremely medical treatments can be extremely effective and changing your diet can help ease the symptoms.

The diet that is presented in this book is not an off the wall diet that was developed to trick you into feeling like you are in control. There is scientific evidence behind it and there is a great deal of research proving that gluten, and foods containing gluten are the number one cause of flares in individuals who have autoimmune disorders.

How Does a Gluten Free Diet Help Reduce Symptoms?

Gluten is a substance that is found in a large variety of foods. Even without an autoimmune disorder, it is proven that gluten causes inflammation in joints and other tissues throughout the body. Combined with an autoimmune diseases, this inflammation can become out of control, leading to a lot of long term damage and a greater feeling of discomfort in those who suffer from an autoimmune disorder.

Why Treatments Are Limited for Autoimmune Disorders

Autoimmune disorders affect different body systems and organs. Over time, it has been difficult to determine the exact burden that autoimmune diseases carry, mostly because studies have not focused on them as single entities, but as a whole. This is because there are so many autoimmune disorders that are considered rare, that it would be difficult to get enough people together to complete accurate scientific studies. Research on various autoimmune diseases have focused mostly on the number of people who have been affected by the diseases, the morbidity of the disease and the financial cost in treating each disorder, rather than finding better treatments for the diseases that are diagnosable.

To give you an idea of how many people are affected by autoimmune disorders in the general population, approximately 50 million people in the United States suffer from some type of autoimmune diseases. This number trumps that of heart disease, which affects approximately 25.5 million people. The worst part is that the prevalence of autoimmune disorders is rising, but there is not much scientific research going into finding a permanent cure, since there are so many diseases and they are each treated in a different fashion.

Autoimmune disorders are considered chronic, or long term disorders that have no cure. Because of this, treatment for each disorder involves lifetime treatment and it is noted that without the proper care, these disorders cause a high incidence of morbidity, disability, mortality and cost approximately $100 Billion dollars each year to treat, and these numbers only cover the United States.

Due to lack of information and lack of community awareness, many patients with autoimmune disorders go undiagnosed. This is because diagnosing one can be extremely challenging. To make matters worse, getting a diagnosis for a chronic autoimmune disease can take years and a lot of embarrassment and labeling along the way. Studies have shown that at least 45 % of the people with autoimmune disorders claim to have been labeled as chronic complainers, hypochondriacs or drug seekers before they received a diagnosis. This is mostly because the treating physician could not determine the cause of the symptoms, since the disease was in its early stages and diagnostic testing could not pick up the markers that trigger the results that doctors typically look for in blood tests.

As you can assume, there are a certain diseases that are more likely to cause a higher incidence of death than others if treatment plans are not followed, or a diagnosis is not reached. While these diseases have increased in incidence, the number of deaths associated with these disorders has decreased dramatically since 1995.

There is a lot about autoimmune diseases that are still unknown, but medical science has developed enough to manage the conditions and extend life expectancy for many of those affected.

Pathogenesis

The immune system is initially designed to work with a wide balance of factors that respond to a variety of foreign threats. These threats are typically things like harmful bacteria, viruses, cancer cells and other illness inducing agents, while maintaining a self-tolerance.

In a small percentage of people, the balance is disrupted. The immune system loses its ability to tolerate certain types of cells in the body. The resulting autoimmunity can need to development of autoimmune diseases. Typically, an autoimmune disease involves damage to specific organs, tissues, or cells. However, there is no limit to what an out of control immune system can do. Over time, almost any body system can become affected and it can develop into what doctors call "multi-organ involvement."

Organ Specific Diseases

Organ specific diseases, such as thyroiditis, type 1 diabetes, MS, and inflammatory bowel disease do exist. They do not spread any further than the specified organ and the inflammation is directed specifically to the target organ.

Organ specific autoimmune diseases can differ greatly according to whether the disease is mediated through autoantibodies, autoreactive T-cells, or a combination of the two.

It is important to note, that just because a lab value returns with an autoantibody does not mean that you actually have the disease. Some autoantibodies are found in people who have no evidence of an autoimmune disease. Also, the autoantibodies can be present years before the disease actually develops. Because there is a high incidence of autoimmune response in every human being, this leads scientists to believe that there is more to the development of autoimmune diseases than simple laboratory values. This means that other factors, either internal or external must be involved in the development of an autoimmune disorder.

Risk Factors

When it comes to the development of an autoimmune disorder, there are many factors that researchers have found that leave a person predisposed to developing an autoimmune disorder.

Genetic Factors

Genetic Factors have been found to play a huge roll in whether a person is susceptible to developing an autoimmune disorder. IN general, autoimmune diseases typically affect those with a family history of the disorder, which means that there is some incidence of inheritance.

Currently, there are at least 68 different genetic risk factors that have been proven in scientific studies, however the problem lies with the fact that the genetic studies only prove that there is an increased risk of developing an autoimmune disorder. It does not have to be the same exact autoimmune disorder that was exhibited by the family member who passed on the gene.

Environmental Factors

Environmental factors have proven their role in the development of autoimmune diseases. The exact triggers and how their interactions with current genetic predisposition cause the disorder are not yet known. Many of the environmental risk factors that have been located are infections agents, stress, hormones, cigarette smoking and drug use.

Infectious Agents

Another important factor in the development of an autoimmune disorder is an infectious agent. Studies have been conducted on various animal models that have provided some of the best evidence of infectious agents triggering autoimmune disease. During these studies, researchers theorized that the immune response triggered by antigens of microorganisms that resemble self-antigens, a theory that they are currently referring to as molecular mimicry.

A second theory is that autoimmunity is induced by a mechanism that is known as the bystander effect. This is where the invading microorganism directly damages the active infection that directly exposes antigens to the immune system.

The typical diseases that are associated by infection as the main problem is an infectious agents are:

Multiple sclerosis
Type 1 diabetes
Rheumatoid arthritis
Systemic lupus
Fibromyalgia
Myasthenia gravis
Guillain-Barre syndrome

The microorganisms that are typically to blame for the activation of these diseases are viral. These diseases include:

Epstein-Barr
Hepatitis C
Parvo Virus
Cytmealovirus

Stress

In several studies, stress was also proven to be a trigger for autoimmune diseases. Thes studies have been conducted in humans and animals. Stress has a dramatic effect on the immune system and can cause the immune system to react in a lot of different ways. Stress also has the capability to cause alteration in the way that the immune system moderates itself. As a result, scientists and researchers have deducted that stress may be an active factor in the development of abnormal immune responses. There are some autoimmune diseases that are more likely to be triggered by stress, such as systemic lupus, rheumatoid arthritis and fibromyalgia. While scientific studies have shown marked depreciation of the disease, the scientific studies have lacked the power to determine how much stress can actually affect the predomininace of autoimmune diseases.

Reproductive Hormones

Reproductive hormones and the metabolites and receptors that are involved in their regulation and lifespan may cause an immunoregulation response. Their roles in the maturation of lymphocytes, activation and synthesis of antibodies and cytokines.

The reason scientists and researchers feel that sex hormones are a factor in autoimmunity dysregulation are that individuals with autoimmune diseases have some form of hormone deficit. Also, in women, most flares occur around the time of menstruation or during pregnancy. However, more research is needed to determine how much of a role reproductive hormones play in the manifestation of an autoimmune disease, or the advancement of the disease itself.

Cigarette Smoking

Studies have shown that those who smoke, or are exposed to cigarette smoke are at greater risk of developing an autoimmune disease. The most common autoimmune diseases that are triggered by smoking, or exposure to cigarette smoke are rheumatic diseases, systemic lupus and thyroiditis. It is uncertain why cigarette smoke triggers the autoimmune response in so many people.

Other Risk Factors

In 2014, over $2.4 million dollars in funding was provided to research studies that were looking into the environmental exposures that could cause the development of autoimmune diseases. In addition to what we have listed above, other environmental factors were found, including:

Exposure to crystalline silica
Exposure to solvents
Exposure to UV Radiation

There were also research studies done into the timing of exposure, for example:

Fetal perinatal
Prepuberty
Puberty
Adult
Various ages in adult hood

Unfortunately these studies did not yield a great deal of information.

Chapter 3: General Characteristics

Each autoimmune disease has a very distinct entity with its own signs and symptoms. Many autoimmune diseases will share some common characteristics, including female preponderance, similar symptoms profiles, and difficulty in diagnosing the disorder. The importance of taking the, and providing a full physical history and physical examination is detrimental to the diagnosis.

Autoimmune diseases have a prominent gender bias. Women account for at least 80% of the cases of autoimmune diseases across the globe. Certain diseases have an even higher incidence of developing in females. For example Hashimoto's Thyroiditis prefers females 95% of the time.

Just like any other scientific fact, there are exceptions to the rule. For example, type 1 diabetes, ulcerative colitis and Guillan-Barre syndrome and psoriasis are more common in men than they are in women.

Female Predominance of Autoimmune Disorders and Fibromyalgia

Disease	Approximate Female to Male Ratio
Hashimoto's Thyroiditis	10: 1
Sjogren Syndrome	9: 1
Systemic Lupus Erythemoatosus	9:1
Antipohsphlipid Syndrome – Secondary	9.1
Primary Biliary Cirrhosis	9:1
Graves' Disease	7:1
Scleroderma	3:1
Rheumatoid Arthritis	2.5:1
Antiphosphlipid syndrome – primary	2: 1
Multiple Sclerosis	2: 1
Myastheina Gravis	2:1
Fibromyalgia	2: 1

Symptom Profiles of Auto Immune Diseases

The symptom profiles for autoimmune disorders contain a lot of shared characteristics. The most common symptoms include low grad fever, dizziness and an overall feeling of not being well. They also include a variety of other symptoms that come and go over time. There are periods of remission, flares and just not feeling well at all.

Autoimmune Disorders and Difficulty with Diagnosis

There is evidence mounding up that it is extremely difficult to diagnose autoimmune diseases. It is proven that a large number of patients who eventually end up with a diagnosis of an autoimmune disorder are typically marked as hypochondriacs or complainers at the start of their medical journey. Many people give up before receiving a diagnosis, others persist until they find a doctor that will listen to them and take their complaints seriously.

The true shock value is that it can take as long as 2 to 5 years to diagnose an autoimmune disease, and by then, most patients have given up and sentenced themselves to a life of dealing with their symptoms on their own. Also, during this extensive period of time, the symptoms can begin to affect many different body organs, making it difficult for a physician to determine what disease it is and how far it has progressed. This typically results in patients seeing multiple specialists before they are actually treated for their disorder, even after a doctor believes that something is wrong.

Importance of History and Physical Examination in Diagnosis

The best way to determine whether or not a patient has an autoimmune disorder is to do a complete history and physical examination, as well as a full battery of blood tests. A responsible doctor will prompt patients about symptoms that patients may have, but do not think it is important enough to tell their doctor about. They should also ask about any family history of an autoimmune disorder.

Chapter 4: Do You Have An Autoimmune Disease?

If you're not sure whether or not you have an autoimmune disease, check out some of these common signs:

- Difficulty concentrating or focusing (brain fog)
- Chronic fatigue
- Weight loss or weight gain for unknown reasons
- Several miscarriages
- Abnormal hair loss or white patches on your skin
- Constant dry eyes and dry mouth
- Abdominal pain, cramping, bloating or frequent diarrhea
- Numbness or tingling in feet and hands
- Joint pain and/or swelling
- Feeling sick or achy a lot of the time
- Heat intolerance
- Recurrent skin rashes or sun-sensitivity

Even if you have several of these symptoms, do not assume you have an autoimmune disease unless you've checked with a doctor. Sometimes, these symptoms can be caused by other problems unrelated to an autoimmune disease, so do not automatically jump to the conclusion or attempt to self-diagnose.

In order to ensure that you are actually suffering from an autoimmune disorder, your doctor will need to run a series of blood tests and take a full physical examination. It may take some time to diagnose the disorder, and the diagnosis may not be immediate. This is because your doctor must ensure that you have an autoimmune disorder before you are prescribed medication. This is because the medication for autoimmune disorders can be extremely dangerous if you have a different condition, or an underlying condition that does not react well to the medication your doctor would typically prescribe.

What Body Parts Does an Autoimmune Disease Effect?

Since autoimmune diseases develop when the immune system attacks healthy body cells, autoimmune diseases can affect every area of the body in some way. These affects can include:

- Glands
- Nerves
- Brain
- Muscles
- Skin
- Heart
- Kidney

- Uterus
- Eyes
- Mouth
- Intestines
- Pancreas
- Joints
- Lung
- And more

It's critical to take the time to figure out how to help yourself relieve the symptoms of the disease. Consulting with a health practitioner for an accurate diagnosis is the first step. Then, you can effectively treat symptoms and take back control of your life forever.

Common Treatments for Autoimmune Diseases

This list autoimmune disorders very similar baseline symptoms, many of them are treated it a similar fashion. Key component in any the immune disorder is to stop the immune system from seeing the body as its own enemy. To do this, doctors use a wide variety of treatments, including steroids.

The reason that steroids are used is because they are known for helping the body to heal itself faster, and to help keep the immune system in proper working order. Steroids are typically combined with a wide variety of other medications, depending on the type of disorder you are facing.

The initial treatment of steroids may be given in intravenous form, which has been proven extremely effective in providing almost instant relief. Other forms of direct treatment are injections, or oral steroids that provide relief from the inflammation, and slow the immune system response down dramatically.

Steroids may be prescribed intermittently or permanently, depending on your condition. Some conditions only require you to take a steroid shot once per month, which is extremely convenient, especially compared to the other alternatives that are available.

Another common treatment for autoimmune disorders is a serious change in diet. There are many different ingredients that can make cause sensitivities to your autoimmune disorder. Many people have found that changing their diet on a long term basis is more effective than taking the medication that is prescribed for the disorder. They also find that it is less expensive to change their diet than it is to buy the expensive medications that standard physicians prescribe for these disorders.

Chapter 5: Cancer as an Autoimmune Disorder

Modern science and research have found a direct correlation between the creation of an autoimmune disorder and the various disroders that are classified as cancerous. Researchers at George Washington University in Washinton DC, located a direct link between autoimmune diseases and cancer cell reactions. They have also proven that both diseaases cause identical cellular responses and cause the body to release the same cell destruction inhibitors.

You may wonder how one can compare cancer to an autoimmune disorder, but in truth, cancer has all of the markers of an autoimmune disorder and causes the same autoimmune response.

Cancer Verses Autoimmune Disorder

Even though cancer and autoimmune disorders share a common ground, they do have some differences.

Autoimmune diseases cause an abnormal reaction to healthy cells that are already existent in the body, whereas cancer cells are attacked because they are abnormal.

Essentially, in cancer, the body's own cells change, alter, or reproduce themselves at astronomical rates. The body then sends immune cells to fight off the excess cells that are building up in the body. Over time, the immune system becomes weak and the cancerous cells are located by a doctor.

Having an Autoimmune Disease Does Not Mean You Have Cancer

Comparing cancer to an autoimmune disorder does serve a purpose. However, before we dive further into this concept, we want to point out that having an autoimmune disorder does not automatically mean that you have cancer. It does however mean that the two types of disorders have a similar reaction in the body, and since most people have a basic understanding of the way that cancer works, it is a great starting point to learning exactly how autoimmune diseases work inside the body. It also brings an interesting new twist into all of the ways the body's immune system can go off kilter and cause serious and dangerous issues inside the body without warning.

The discovery of the similarities between cancer and autoimmune diseases increases the chances of developing new treatments for both, and also increases the chance of developing a cure for multiple diseases in the near future.

Chapter 6: All About Inflammation

Inflammation is not a synonym for infection, even though many people think that it is. Inflammation is a response to infection, but they are not related biologically. Some microorganisms like bacteria, viruses, can cause infection causing inflammation. Inflammation is the body's response against any external or internal stimuli to fight against:

- Injury
- minimize the cell damage
- remove the invaders
- damaged cells and tissues
- Start the healing process

Although both these words are strongly correlated (and inflammation usually results after an infection), it is important to understand the difference.

As infection is usually followed by an inflammation, so sometimes it is misinterpreted with infection. Sometimes, inflammation can occur without an infection as in autoimmune disorders like rheumatoid arthritis in which body misreads its own cells as foreign invaders or damaged or abnormal cells and starts killing them, even if they are perfectly healthy cells.

Without inflammation, progressive destruction can be dangerous and compromises the survival of the infected individual. On the other hand, chronic inflammation can lead to some diseases like rheumatoid arthritis, hay fever, atherosclerosis and even cancer.

Causes of Inflammation

Factors that can cause inflammation are infectious microorganisms, physical and chemical agents, inappropriate response of the immune system and tissue death. The most common cause of the inflammation are microorganisms, bacteria and viruses. Viruses cause inflammation by entering and killing the host cells, and bacteria releasing endotoxins inside the host body that leads to the inflammation.

Physical trauma, frostbite, radiations, corrosive acids, alkalis and toxins, and burns damage the body cells and can trigger the inflammation process. Another important cause, as mentioned earlier, of inflammation is the misleading autoimmune response of the body. Inflammation can also begin when cells or tissues in certain areas of the body start dying because of the lack of oxygen and nutrients. This situation usually arises when certain areas of body are deprived of blood flow.

Classic Signs of Inflammation

Although Latin terms are widely used in the medical field, especially in the Western medicine, English, being the most influencing international language is taking over now.

A modern English acronym for describing classical symptoms of pain is 'PRISH'. However, the classical Latin based terms of inflammation has been around for over 2000 years.

- Dolor: This Latin term is for 'pain'
- Calor: A Latin term for 'heat'
- Rubor: This Latin term stands for 'redness'
- Tumor: Tumor is the Latin terms for 'swelling'
- Functio Laesa: This Latin term means 'injured function', which can also be described as 'loss of function'

The above inflammation signs are only relevant when inflammation occurs on or very close to skin. If inflammation occurs in deep internal organ, only a few signs of inflammation can be detected. Some internal organs might not have attached nerve endings nearby, so there might not be pain associated with such inflammations as in some cases of pneumonia (inflammation of the lung). Pneumonia causes pain sensation when pneumonia inflammation pushes alongside parietal pleura.

Blood Tests to Detect Inflammation

- Erythrocyte sedimentation test (ESR).
- C Reactive Protein Test
- Plasma viscosity test

Chapter 7: Major Components of Inflammation

There are two types of inflammation: Acute and chronic inflammation

Acute Inflammation
Immediately starts after an injury or a stimulus attack and quickly becomes severe. This is the body's first response to any external or internal stimuli and typically lasts only for a few days, but sometimes it may persists for weeks or even months until the injury heals.

Process of Acute Inflammation
Acute inflammatory process involves two types of changes: the vascular changes and cellular changes.

Vascular Changes
When any cell or tissue of the body is injured, vasoconstriction occurs in the injured area and small blood vessels in the damaged area constricts immediately. After this transient phase of vasoconstriction, which is considered

less important to the inflammatory response, vasodilatation begins, which dilates the blood vessels and increases the blood flow to the damaged area. The phase of vasodilatation lasts for 15 minutes to several hours.

Vasodilatation is followed by increased permeability of blood vessels. Usually, walls of blood vessels only allow the passage of smaller water and salt molecules, but following an injury, the permeability of blood vessels is increased. Now the exudate, the protein rich fluid can exit into the extra cellar fluid of the tissues. As the acute phase continues the exudate exits into the tissues, clotting factors present in the exudate prevent spread of the microorganisms throughout the body. Antibodies present in the exudate try to destroy and kill the invading microorganisms.

As exudate and other fluids continue to leak out of the blood vessels, the blood flow becomes slower and white blood cells, or WBCs, start to pile up in the center of the blood vessel, so that they can flow closer to the vessel wall. In later part of this phase, the WBCs start adhering to the blood vessel walls, which is their first step towards emigration into the extra cellular space of the injured tissues.

Cellular Changes
The accumulation of WBCs at the site of injury is the most important feature of the acute inflammation. Most important cells in this phase are neutrophils, certain phagocytes that engulf the injury causing microbes and clear the cellular debris formed because of the injury.

Neutrophils, a type of white blood cell, having some cell destroying enzymes and proteins are the main phagocytes involved in ingesting the bacteria/viruses in the acute inflammation process. When a minor injury or tissue damage occurs, the supply of neutrophils can be obtained from the circulating blood, but when extensive tissue damage occurs, massive amounts of neutrophils, even some in immature form, are released from the bone marrow, the place where neutrophils are generated. Migration of the neutrophils to the injury site causes swelling of the injured area and released mediators cause pain sensations.

To perform their functions, neutrophils need to exit from the walls of the blood vessels and to move towards the injury site. This movement is facilitated by a concentration gradient formed by the substances which are diffused out from the area of tissue damage. The substances released from the injury site that create the concentration gradient are named as chemotactic factors, and the one-way movement of the neutrophils along the gradient is called chemotaxis.

A huge number of neutrophils reach the infection or injury site, sometimes the migration of neutrophils only need an hour or half to reach the injury site. After neutrophils reach to the injury area, inflammation usually takes 24-28 hours to begin. After this, monocytes, which is a type of WBC, joins the injury site and mature into cell eating macrophages. Macrophages become more evident after some days or even after some weeks of the injury. Macrophages are the hallmark of the chronic inflammation.

Leukocytes are believed to have a role in the initiation and maintenance of the inflammatory process. Leukocytes must be reached from their usual place in blood to the injury site to perform their functions. Therefore, some mechanism exists for the migration of leukocytes from blood to the injury site. The process of the migration of the leukocytes is called extravasation.

Some leukocytes act as phagocytes and engulf invading bacteria, viruses and cellular debris. Some leukocytes are known to release some enzymatic granules that destroy the invaded microbes. Leukocytes are known to release meditators for initiating and maintaining the inflammatory process. Generally, granulocytes mediate the acute inflammation, whereas chronic inflammation is mediated by leukocytes and monocytes. The acute inflammation phase needs continuous stimulation to move on, but the inflammatory mediators have short life and are depleted in the tissues after removal of the stimulus, as there is no continuous stimulus, so acute inflammation stops.

Plasma Cascade event
- The complement system, once activated produces a series of chemical events that promote chemotaxis, agglutination and opsonization and produces MAC (membrane attack complex).

- The fibrinolysis system plays its role by opposing the coagulation process and generates several inflammatory mediators.

- The coagulation system produces a protective layer around the injury site.

- The kinn system releases some proteins, which then sustain the vasodilatation process and some other inflammatory effects.

Chemical Mediators of Inflammation

The inflammatory response begins after an injury, but the chemical mediators released following the injury help to start the cellular and vascular changes that are described above. These chemical mediators are primarily obtained from the blood plasma, WBCs, mast cells, epithelial lining of the vessels, platelets and from the damaged or injured cells.

Histamine is one of the most known chemical mediators released from the cell during the inflammation, and believed to have a role in vasodilatation and increasing permeability of blood vessels. Histamines are the first mediator that is released immediately following the injury.

Lysosomal compounds that are released from neutrophils also increase permeability of the blood vessels. Various cytokines released from the cells play a role in chemotactic and inflammatory processes. Prostaglandins belong to a group of fatty acids and have a role in increasing permeability of the blood vessels.

Prostaglandins help in platelet aggregation and causes pain and fever during inflammation. Prostaglandins are produced from the arachidonic acid pathway just like leukotrienes.

Chapter 8: Events That Occur After Acute Inflammation

Healing: In this process, the cells that are capable of regeneration start healing. Different cells have different healing capabilities. After the inflammation, some cells regenerate very quickly e.g. epithelial cells.

The others cannot regenerate quickly e.g. the liver cells cannot reproduce very quickly, but they can be stimulated to regenerate. Unfortunately, some cells cannot regenerate. The tissue structure needs to be simple enough to be reconstructed. Think about the regeneration of the simple structure of the skin and the complex structure of the kidney, as being a simple structure, the skin can regenerate itself easily and quickly, but for kidney, it is very difficult to reconstruct itself after the injury.

Failure to regenerate in some injury cases can lead to other diseases. When the liver cells are damaged as in cirrhosis, due to abnormal regeneration of the tissue the previous cirrhosis now can lead to hemorrhaging and even to death.

Repair: Repairing of the damaged tissue occurs when there is a major damage to the tissue, or the original structure of the tissue cannot be regained as it was before the injury. Some injuries and damages result in the formation of a fibrous scar.

Epithelial cells form new blood vessels in the injured area via repair process, and fibroblasts cells from a network of loose connective tissue around the injury site. This delicate vasculature is called granulation tissue. New blood vessels start working after establishing a network in the healing area, and collagen tissue produced by fibroblasts provides mechanical strength to the regenerated tissue.

Finally, a dense packed scar of collagen is formed. The scar looks smaller than the tissue it replaces. This scar can cause distortion and contraction of the tissue. When a scar is formed in the intestine issue, the scar can distort the tubular structure of intestine to be obstructed because of narrowing of the tissue. The most dangerous cases of scarring occurs because of severe traumatic injury or burns.

Suppuration

Suppuration is the process of formation of pus at the site of injury when the removal of inflammatory debris is not easily possible. Pus is a thick and viscous fluid, which mostly consists of damaged and necrotic cells, dead bacteria or viruses, neutrophils, macrophages and the exudate liquid leaked from the blood vessels. Staphylococcus and streptococcus infections, the pus forming bacteria, are the main cause behind pus formation. Once pus formation starts in a tissue, it is surrounded by a membrane and give rise to a structure known as abscess.

Treatment of abscess is very difficult as it is not easily accessible to antibiotic agents and antibodies. Sometimes abscess needs a surgical procedure to remove it, while sometimes the abscess bursts own its own after a certain time period, e.g. a boil bursts in this way. After the bursting of the abscess, tissue is replaced with the help of healing process.

Diseases/Conditions that can Cause Acute Inflammation
- Acute sinusitis
- A Blow
- Acute bronchitis
- Sore throat or cold/ flu
- Intense exercise
- Acute appendicitis
- Acute dermatitis
- Any cut/scratch on skin
- Acute tonsillitis
- Acute meningitis
- Infected growing toenail

Chapter 9: Process Of Chronic Inflammation

Chronic inflammation is a long-term inflammation and can stay for several days, weeks
and even for years. Chronic inflammation can occur:

- When the acute inflammatory response fails to remove the causative agent of the inflammation
- A low intensity chronic irritant that persists for long time
- Because of the hyperactive response of immune system against its own cells
- Sometimes as an independent process

Some very dangerous and disabling diseases like rheumatoid arthritis, tuberculosis and chronic lung disease are characterized by chronic inflammation. Chronic inflammation can begin when some viruses and bacteria resist the host defense mechanism and are able to stay for longer duration in the infected tissue.

Some examples of such infectious agents include certain fungi, metazoal parasites and protozoa. Other causes that brought in chronic inflammation are those foreign materials that are not removed by enzymatic breakdown or via phagocytosis. Such materials include inhaled silica dust and the material that gets in the wounds e.g. metal or wood splinters.

The stimulus to chronic inflammation in the autoimmune diseases is the normal component of the body, but the problem is that the immune system has become sensitive to it. An autoimmune reaction produces some inflammatory diseases like rheumatoid arthritis.

Presence of plasma cells, lymphocytes and macrophages at inflammation site is the true indication of chronic inflammation. These cells are obtained from the circulatory blood with the help of chemotactic factors. The key components of the chronic inflammation are macrophage that leads to tissue destruction and loss of functionality of the involved tissue.

A typical chronic inflammation is granulomatous inflammation. This inflammation is characterized by the formation of granulomas, a collection of modified macrophages surrounded by lymphocytes. Tuberculosis is a classic example of granulomatous inflammation.

Diseases Associated with Chronic Inflammation
- Chronic sinusitis
- Chronic Active hepatitis
- Chronic periodontitis
- Chronic peptic ulcer
- Asthma

- Tuberculosis
- Crohn's disease
- Rheumatoid arthritis
- Ulcerative colitis

Comparison of Acute and Chronic Inflammation

Characteristic	Acute Inflammation	Chronic Inflammation
Causative Agents	Harmful pathogens or injurious agents	Certain pathogens that resist host defense mechanism, and are capable of long stay at the injury site. Hyperactive responses of immune system
Main Cell Types Involved	Mainly neutrophils and basophils in inflammatory responses, and eosinophils against worm and parasitic inflammations, and macrophages and monocytes generally	Plasma cells, lymphocytes, macrophages and fibroblasts
Onset	Immediately after the injury	After the failure of chronic inflammation to remove the causative agent of injury, after certain pathogens and because of autoimmune diseases

Mediators	Vasoactive amines and eicosanoids	Hydrolytic enzymes, growth factors and reactive oxygen species
Duration	Short, usually lasts for a few days	From several months to years
Outcomes	Resolution of inflammation, development of abscess or leads to chronic inflammation	Destruction of the tissue, formation of scar, death of tissues or cells

Inflammation and Innate Immunity

Innate immunity is a type of immunity that we get from nature at the time of birth. Innate immunity is contrary to the adaptive immunity that we get after an infection or through vaccination. However, innate immunity, we get from nature, is nonspecific, while the adaptive immunity is specific for different diseases.

Example of Polio and Adaptive Immunity

During childhood, children are vaccinated for poliovirus. The polio vaccine produces antibodies against the poliovirus in the blood so that if children are exposed to poliovirus, that already circulating antibodies in blood will kill the invading poliovirus and in this way saves children from getting the polio.

This is how adaptive immunity is developed and how it helps us in protecting against certain lifelong disabling and dangerous diseases. Inflammation is generally considered a mechanism of innate immunity.

Children are vaccinated for a large number of diseases early in life. They require booster shots intermittently thoroughout their life to maintain immunity and to help them become immune to new strains of the virus as it mutates, attempting to survive.

Chapter 10: Inflammation and Pain

When anybody gets inflammation, it often hurts that person. People having inflammation feel moderate to severe pain, stiffness, discomfort and distress based on the severity of inflammation. Inflammation often causes steady and constant pain referred to as ache. Inflammatory pain is unique and distinct that only be best described by the person who experience it. This pain can be acute or chronic. Generally, inflammation causes pain because swelling in the inflamed areas pushes against the walls of the sensory nerve endings that are sensitive to stretch or touch.

Visceral Pain

Visceral pain is a type of nociceptive pain, and is felt down in the body in the internal organs and main cavities like heart, kidney, spleen, bladder, ovaries, uterus, and liver. It is very difficult to locate the visceral pain. The nociceptive receptors sense inflammation, ischemia and tissue stretch. Colicky sensation and cramping pain are typical examples of visceral pain.

Somatic Pain

This pain is also a nociceptive pain. The pain sensation is usually felt is bones, joints, ligaments and on the skin. Musculoskeletal pain is also characterized as somatic pain. Pain receptors for somatic pain are sensitive to muscle stretch, vibration, temperature and inflammation.

Nociceptive Pain

Specific receptors set are activated to feel this pain. These receptors are sensitive to temperature, vibration, stretch and certain chemicals that are released after injury of the cells. The meaning of the word Nociceptive is 'causing or reacting to pain'. The cause of the pain is usually from outside of the nervous system and then nervous system reacts or responds to it.

Risk factors for Inflammation

- Toxic foods: High processed carb and sugar diet, high intake of fatty foods, conventionally raised beef meat, all these food are associated with increased risk of inflammation.

- Excessive Intake of Omega 6: Omega 6 fats are the precursors for eicosanoids, cells involved in the inflammation. So taking high amounts of Omega 6 fats can be dangerous.

- Less Intake of Omega 3: Omega 3 are known as the precursors of anti-inflammatory eicosanoids, that are very important component of the inflammatory process, so taking low amount of Omega 3 means less precursors of anti-inflammatory eicosanoids.

- Chronic Stress: Our life is stressful these days. Extensive workloads, politics, work commitments, heavy bills, exercise for which we cannot find time, instability and growing unemployment, multi-factorial approach towards our daily lives, all these go on increasing. All these become very difficult to handle. There are great chances that your body will get a physiological inflammatory response because of these emotional stresses.

- Inadequate Sleep: Inadequate or poor sleep is linked to elevated risk for inflammation. Disturbed sleep patterns or not getting proper sleep is a chronic and widely growing problem in the developed nations. We usually go to bed late, get up early or spend a lot of amount on our smart devices in the little time we get for sleep.

- Poor Gut Health: A larger part of our immune system is integrated in the gut system. When you have a poor health of your gut, it means your inflammatory response is not good enough.

- Too Busy Life: When we are always using our computer, smartphone for checking emails, communicating people or entertaining, indirectly we are putting our brain and body under great stress. We are humans, not computers or machines. So our body needs a down time. Busy lifestyles of today can disturb our immune system and so inflammatory response.

- Not Enjoying Nature: These days we spend our time inside rooms, buses, trains, cities and do not go towards parks, wildlife zoos, open airs to enjoy nature. Spending sometime enjoying nature can have positive effect on our body

- Sedentary Lifestyle: Today, because of technology-oriented lifestyle, we are 'unknowingly' leading sedentary life, and lack of movement and activity is directly linked to low graded systemic inflammation. We have forgotten how to walk on foot; instead, we always use automobiles for going here and there. We do not have time for exercise either.

- Over Activity: Some people work and ran too much and do not give their bodies some downtime to recover. People that work out a lot without allowing body to recover fully can become chronically inflamed.

Pain is a normal response to inflammation and injury. Typically, pain is a great gage to register when something is wrong and helps you and your doctor to locate the origin of the injury or problem that you are facing healthwise.

While it may not seem like a helpful tool, it is actually an amazing diagnositic tool for your doctor to gage where an injury or disease progression has developed. Even though you may not think that pain is a good for you, a little bit of pain can help diagnostically and can help in the healing process.

Chapter 11: Possible Treatments for Inflammation

All healthcare professional, allied health workers and patients must remember, as described earlier in this book, that inflammation is one of the most important aspect of healing process. Sometimes it becomes mandatory to reduce the inflammation, but sometimes it is not required at all.

Anti-Inflammatory Drugs
Non-Steroidal Anti Inflammatory Drugs (NSAIDS)

NSAIDS are used to reduce the pain associated with the inflammation. NSAIDS block the cyclooxygenase enzymes, which are known to produce prostaglandins, the pain causing mediators. By blocking synthesis of prostaglandins, the pain sensation either can be eliminated or reduced significantly.

Examples of NSAIDS Drugs: Naproxen, Naproxen sodium, ibuprofen, aspirin

A word of Caution about NSAIDS: NSAIDS should not be used regularly or long term without supervision of the physician. Stomach ulcers and life threatening hemorrhage is associated with long-term use of NSAIDS. These drugs can also worse the asthma symptoms and increase the kidney damage. Except aspirin, other NSAIDS drugs are associated to myocardial infarction and stroke.

Acetaminophen (Paracetamol, Tylenol): Acetaminophen though can decrease the pain associated with an inflammation, but cannot help in reducing the inflammation. Acetaminophen is a great drug for those who only want to get rid of the pain, but want to inflammation process go on.

Immune Selective Anti-Inflammatory Derivatives:
IMULAN Bio Therapeutics, LLC, formulated this class of anti-inflammatory drug. Some studies have clearly showed that these drugs have anti-inflammatory properties. The mechanism of action of this class changes the activation and migration of those cells of the immune system that proliferate the inflammatory response. Still, this class is being used in animals, but it is believed that soon these drugs will be available for human use.

Corticosteroids
Corticosteroids are naturally produced steroidal hormones that are produced in the outer portion of the adrenal gland. Now, they are formulated in the laboratories and are added in the medicines.

Corticosteroid drugs have anti-inflammatory action, they block the release of phospholipids, because of this blockage, and a number of inflammatory mechanisms are weakened.

There are two main classes of corticosteroids.

Glucocorticoids:

When we are under stress, our body synthesizes glucocorticoids. They are believed to have a role in the metabolism of proteins, fats and carbohydrates. Synthetic corticosteroids are used for the inflammation of many immune disorders like arthritis, asthma, hepatitis, etc. Topical formulations of glucocorticoids may be prescribed for the inflammation of eyes, skin, lungs and nose.

Mineralocorticoids:

This class of corticosteroids is known for regulating water and salt balance in our body. Drugs having mineralocorticoids are used for cerebral salt wasting and in the patients having adrenal insufficiency.

Corticosteroids side effects are associated with the dosage forms being used and the frequency of use of these drugs. The chances of developing side effects are more likely with oral corticosteroids compared to inhalers, injectable or dermatological preparations

Inhaled corticosteroids if used in the long run for treating asthma may raise the risk of developing oral thrush. Rinsing the mouth with fresh water after every application of the inhaler might be beneficial in this regard. Glucocorticoids use can lead to Cushion's Syndrome, whereas hypertension can develop with mineralocorticoids use.

Certain Foods/Herbs Having Anti-Inflammatory Response

- Turmeric (Curcuma longa): This plant belongs to ginger family. Research is in progress to find out some benefits of this plant to treat Alzheimer disease, rheumatoid arthritis and some other inflammatory disorders.

- Cannabis: Cannabis contains cannabichromene a chemical that is believed to have some anti-inflammatory properties.

- Ginger: Ginger is both used as a condiment and drug. Since long time, ginger has been used as carminative agent. It is being used since hundreds of years a medicine against dyspepsia, colic and constipation and to reduce arthritis pain.

- Hyssop Hyssopus: This plant belongs to plant family Lamiaceae. It is also used in the coloration of some spirits. This herb is mixed with other herbs like liqourice and is used in the treatment of lung diseases and some inflammations. Be careful, as the oils of these herbs are very dangerous.

- Harpagophytum procumbens: Other names for this herb are wood spider, devil's claw and it is known as grapple plant. It is indigenous to South Africa and resembles to sesame plants. This herb is believed to have sedative, diuretic and analgesic properties.

- Shiitake mushrooms: Having high molecular weight polysaccharides, these Asian mushrooms are known to improve overall immune system.

- Chia Seeds: They are rich in Omega 3 fats and fight against inflammation

- Probiotic and Enzyme Salad: This salad is known to promote gut flora and digestive system. It also helps in detoxification and fighting against inflammation.

- Blueberries: Blueberries contain high amounts of anti-oxidant agents. They are very delicious, healthy and anti-inflammatory food items.

Chapter 12: What is an Anti-Inflammatory Diet?

When you are looking for a diet plan that can help the issues that you are having with inflammation, than the ant-inflammatory diet might be the one for you. This diet is different from others in many ways, not just because of the fact that it does not have a fancy name like some of the others.

While most diet plans will concentrate on helping followers to lose weight and to manage a host of health issues, this particular diet plan is just meant to deal with the issues that come with inflammation in the joints. Sure, you will be able to see some weight loss and increases in your overall health, but these are more because of the foods that you will be eating and those that you will be avoiding rather than because of the diet in particular.

An inflammatory diet plan is less of a diet and more of a new way to eat for the rest of your life that can help with the issues that can come with inflammation in the joints. This is a whole group of diets that all work towards the same goal of helping you to feel better and move around much easier. There is a lot of websites, books, and other information that is available on this diet that can help you to be successful on this diet plan and each of the plans that fit under the name will have a slightly different spin on how you should go about achieving the end results.

Many nutritionists agree that a diet that fits under this heading can be amazing for your overall health, even if you are not currently suffering from the pain of inflammation. Some other diseases that may be prevented by following one of these diets include soothing your arthritic joints, reducing your blood pressure and blood cholesterol, manage any current and existing heart conditions that you may have, and reduce your risk of developing heart disease in the future.

Some of these health conditions will be more effectively treated with an eating plan found on this kind of diets, while others may still need some outside treatment. There will need to be more evidence gathered in order to determine how effective this kind of diet plan will be with some of the outside health conditions.

The first question that you may have about this kind of diet is what an anti-inflammatory diet is. This is basically a diet plan that is meant to health the body health any constant and consistent inflammation within it on its own. This will be done by monitoring the types of foods that you are consuming in order to ward off the inflammation.

There are several different types of diets that can fit under this heading and all of them have shown great results in helping with the inflammation in your body. In addition, if you are able to reduce the inflammation that you are feeling inside your body, this could lead to other health conditions being prevented or managed.

According to Russell Greenfield, a professor at the University of North Carolina at Chapel Hill as well as a private practice physician, "It's very clear that inflammation plays a role much more than we thought with respect to certain maladies." As more is known about inflammation and how it can be cured and managed, there may be even more to uncover in the years to come.

There will still need to be more research done, but the preliminaries seem to show that a lot of diseases may be triggered just because of the inflammation that is found in the body. These diseases might include cancer, heart disease, Alzheimer's, and even appendicitis.

Most people do not think of inflammation as more than something that is irritating them and making it difficult to get the things done that they want, but often there is a lot more to it. In some cases, you might not even know that you are dealing with any inflammation at all, which can make it even more of a concern. Some people will have very high levels of inflammation while feeling just fine.

Those who are following the traditional American diet will be eating a lot of foods that have omega-6 fatty acids. These acids are found in the fast foods and processed foods that are so tasty and fit in easily with the busy American lifestyle.

In addition, most Americans are missing out on the rich omega-3 fatty acids that their body needs to stay healthy and which come from supplements or cold water fish. When these two nutrients are not in synch, it will result in inflammation that will just continue to get worse over time.

Many people will wonder what some of the diets may be that would fit under this kind of category. One of the most popular that can be compared to it is the Mediterranean Diet according to Christopher Cannon, a professor of medicine at Harvard Medical School. He is in charge of writing The Complete Idiot's Guide to The Anti-Inflammation Diet. In this book you will be able to find some of the foods and vitamins that are recommended to people who are following one of these diet plans so that they can be more successful and stay on it for the long term.

Andrew Well, a doctor who was educated at Harvard, is the original developer of this kind of diet plan. Well's has long believed that there are foods in the American diet that will cause the inflammation that many people are feeling. A poor diet would lead to this inflammation and it could be treated by changing up the foods that are in the diet. The bad eating habits will need to be changed as soon as possible in order to help prevent many other health issues such as Alzheimer's, cancer, and heart disease.

Some of the things that might influence the inflammation to occur would include the person's diet, their level of physical activity, stress, and some of the environmental toxins that might be around them. When following an anti-inflammatory diet, you will be getting rid of some of the bad foods that are harming your body and substituting good ones that can help reduce inflammation instead.

The overall idea of the anti-inflammation diet is that you will learn how to boost your mental and physical health, make sure that your body always has the energy that it needs, and reduce your risk of getting certain diseases. You will be able to do this by providing your body with the nutrients that it needs including plenty of water, limited animal proteins, healthy fats, and vegetables and fruits that are high in fibers.

One type of protein that is very much encouraged on this diet plan, even though it is considered an animal protein, is fish because of the high amount of omega-3 fatty acids that can do wonders for the inflammation issue.

This diet is based off the person eating somewhere between 2000 to 3000 calories each day. This number will vary depending on several factors such as your activity level, size, and gender. While on this diet, you get about 40 and 50 percent of these calories from the carbs that you consume. Another 30 percent will come from fat and then the last little bit will come from a protein source. It is recommended that you try to mix each of these nutrients into each of your meals.

This kind of diet plan can be considered a spinoff of the Mediterranean Diet, since it has many of the same ideas and this is where Weil got many of his ideas. The two programs are very similar other than a few extras have been added to help with inflammation such as dark chocolate and green tea. The program will ask followers to eat a lot of fresh foods, especially when it comes to the vegetable and fruits that are needed. The nutrients that are found in these produce are great for fighting off cancer as well as some other degenerative diseases. You should also make sure to eat as many omega-3 fatty acids as possible, usually from fish, and avoid fried and fast foods at all time.

While those are kind of general outlines of what you should look out for on the diet, it becomes a little more specific in terms of the dietary guidelines that you should follow. For example, you are not able to just eat any type of carb that you want and expect this kind of diet plan to work for you.

Instead, you need to take a careful look as the carbs that you are consuming and choose the ones that will help you keep the levels of your blood sugar down and steady. This means that you should never pick out carbs that have been processed or have extra sugars in them. Instead, choose the healthier options such as berries, squashes, beans, and whole grains to enjoy while on this diet plan.

Another thing that you will need to cut down on in this diet plan is saturated fat. This would include things like fatty meats, cream, butter, margarine, partially hydrogenated oils, and vegetable shortenings. Your body might have a lot of trouble processing these unhealthy fats so it is better to choose an option that is healthier for your body.

There are a lot of other fats that you can use on this diet plan including avocados, extra virgin olive oil, and omega-3 fatty acids. These omega-3 fatty acids are critical on this diet plan because they have been shown to be effective at reducing inflammation. Cold water fish, such as herring, sardines, and salmon, are the best ways to get your recommended amounts of omega-3s and you should eat these at least twice a week. If this is not possible for you, a supplement should be taken to ensure you are taking in all of the recommended nutrients.

Protein is important on this diet plan as well in order to keep your muscles growing big and strong. You will need to be careful about how you are getting your protein though since many types of meat are not allowed on this diet plan. Some sources of protein that you could consider would be soybeans, some other types of beans, cheese, yogurt, and fish.

This diet plan emphasizes having a lot of color in your diet. The more color that you have, the more likely you are following the diet plan correctly. Colorful produce is a good idea in order to get the great nutrients that your body needs to prevent inflammation. Some great produce to include would be dark greens that are leafy, cruciferous veggies, yellow and orange fruits, tomatoes, and berries. If you are able to, it is recommended that you choose the organic versions of produce in order to avoid pesticides.

Any water that you are drinking while on this diet plan should be purified. Sometimes a few of the toxins that can be found in the water, such as chloramines and chlorine, can be the cause of your inflammation issues. Tea is another great drink option, especially if you are having it instead of coffee. Pick the oolong, green, or white versions of your favorite teas.

Another benefit that you might also enjoy from these kinds of diet plan is that dark chocolate is allowed and red wine. The dark chocolate must be completely plain and have at least 70 percent chocolate content or it is not allowed. The red wine is a good addition if you are dealing with heart disease because the red wine has been known to help assist with that health condition. You should only drink the red wine in moderation though.

The ideas that come with this diet plan are pretty easy to understand. With this diet plan, you will be changing up your eating habits in the hope that you will be able to reduce the pain that comes with inflammation and some other health conditions that may arise in the process.

While it is possible to lose some weight with this diet plan that is not the main reason that people will choose to go on this diet plan. Rather they want to get some relief of their current pain so that they are able to be around for a long time to come. The next chapters will explore this diet plan in a little more depth so that you can start to understand more of what is lying ahead.

Chapter 13: Eating On The Anti-Inflammatory Diet

Before getting started on any diet plan, it is a good idea to learn what foods that you can eat and which ones that you should avoid. Each diet plan is going to be a little different whether it is in the types or amounts of foods that you can eat or even with the times of day that you can eat those foods.

The anti-inflammatory diet is set up in order to help you change your diet so that you are eating foods that prevent and reduce the amount of inflammation that you are having in your body. This can help you to feel better overall as well as help with the prevention of some other diseases in the future. This chapter is devoted to assisting you to understand more about the eating that is required on this diet plan so that you can see the success that you want.

Foods to Eat

To start with are the foods that you are allowed to eat. The first food that is encouraged on this eating plan is foods that have a lot of omega-3 fatty acids. It has been shown in several studies that these kinds of fatty acids are good at reducing the inflammation that may be occurring in your joints and the rest of your body.

This study found that there is a protein receptor in your body that will trigger the pathways for inflammation that is associated with diabetes and obesity. This receptor will bind together the omega-3 fatty acids so that the inflammation in your body will reduce. And according to the University of Maryland Medical Center, you will be able to get a lot of great omega-3 fatty acids from fish.

Some of the best options to get this nutrient include anchovies, shard, smelt, sardines, and salmon. This does not mean that you just have to eat fish all day long to get this fatty acid; you can also try walnuts, pumpkin oil, pumpkin seeds, soybeans, and flaxseed.

Next on the list are foods that have a lot of vitamin C, because this nutrient has also been shown to reduce inflammation of the body according to Professor Block of the University of California. Through studies, it has been shown that vitamin C is able to lower the levels of the C-reactive protein, also known as CRP. This protein is a strong cause of inflammation in the body and is also linked to diabetes and heart disease as
well. This means that if you are able to inhibit the receptor by getting plenty of vitamin C in your diet, you will not only be able to reduce the inflammation issues, you can also reduce other issues such as diabetes and heart disease. Some of the foods that you should add into this diet plan that are high in vitamin C include cantaloupe, apricots, papaya, strawberries, grapefruit, kiwis, and oranges.

Turmeric is starting to become a popular spice for many people who are trying to improve their overall health. This spice seems to be able to do wonders as reducing the amount of inflammation that you have. According to Dr. Art Presser and Dr. Gene Bruno, both from the American Academy of Nutrition, turmeric is used a lot in Eastern cuisine.

Many of those people report that they deal with less inflammation than those who live in other countries. That is because the turmeric contains curcuminoids that are able to help with the prevention of inflammation because they will inhibit several receptors that start the inflammation up in the first place.

Pineapple is another type of food that you might be able to eat in order to reduce the inflammation that you are dealing with on a regular basis. The flesh and the stem will contain an enzyme that is known as bromelain. This enzyme has been shown in several studies to be effective at reducing a variety of inflammation such as the inflammation that occurs from rheumatoid arthritis, inflammation of the sinuses and the veins, and inflammation that occurs after surgery. This enzyme has also been shown in some cases to help with the treatment of inflammation that occurs when you are suffering from carpal tunnel syndrome.

While on one of these types of diets, you should make sure and go for the whole grains. Many dietitians will advocate all of the great benefits that come with eating a variety of whole grains. One way that you can tell if you are eating whole grains is whether they are fluffy or chewy. If they are fluffy, stay away from them and instead find something that is chewier. There are a lot of different grains that will fit into this category including whole wheat or whole grain pastas, brown rice, and even oats and breads.

Fruits and vegetables are extremely important while following this kind of diet plan since they are going to take up the majority of the meals that you will be eating. When choosing fruits, the more color that you can put on your plate the better.

More variety means that you will be getting more nutrition out of your meals as well as antioxidants that your body needs in order to stay healthy and strong while fighting off inflammation. The more colorful fruits and vegetables that you are able to get into your diet the easier it will be to have your body fight off any inflammation that might occur due to different diseases. It is recommended that you consume at least nine servings of these produces during the day while on one of these diet plans.

Eat the right kinds of fats on this kind of diet in order to get the best benefits that you can for fighting with inflammation. To start with, you need to include at least one omega-3 fatty acid into your diet each day and it is preferable if you are able to get this from a fish source. It is also fine to get it from some sort of supplement if you are having difficulties in getting the right kind of foods in your diet. Some options that you can choose are fish oils, flaxseed, and nuts.

While on this diet plan, you will need to make sure to cut out all of the processed foods that you are used to eating. Processed foods are like poison to someone who is dealing with inflammation in their body so it is best to avoid the as much as possible if you would like to increase your overall health. You should cut back as much as possible on some foods such as sugars, refined grains, any processed foods, and trans and saturated fats.

Antioxidants are critical if you are following this kind of diet. These nutrients have been shown to effectively prevent diseases in those who ate them in their diet in addition to reducing their symptoms from inflammation. There are a lot of foods that you can choose from in order to meet this requirement, such as some types of spices, green tea, whole grains, soy, nuts, mushrooms, vegetables, fruits, and extra virgin olive oil. These can all help to prevent the tissue damage that is known to cause inflammation in the joints when they disappear.

The antioxidants that are found in these foods will block the oxygen that is reactive from getting in to the tissue and causing the damage that is known through inflammation. These antioxidants can also help with preventing dementia, cancer, heart disease, and many other health issues.

The idea behind this kind of diet plan is to change your eating and physical habits. You need to have a whole healthy lifestyle in order to improve your overall health; it will not be enough to just go on a diet and hope that it all will work out. You will need to change a lot of things in your life in order to get all of the great benefits that you are hoping for.

In addition to adding in the good diet that comes from an anti-inflammatory diet, you will need to also cut out some of the stress in your life, adopt a daily exercise routine, and make sure that you are staying away from toxins such as smog and tobacco smoke. Doing all of this will do wonders for your body and help you to feel much better.

Foods to Avoid

Now that you have a good idea of the types of foods that your body will need to have while you are on a diet plan like this one, you will now need to learn which foods must be avoided if you want to continue getting the benefits promised in this diet plan. It will not do you any good to eat all of the right foods if you are still including all of the bad foods in your diet at the same time.

Avoiding certain foods while on this diet plan is just as important as anything else that you can do. Here are some of the foods that you should try to avoid as much as possible to get the best benefits from this kind of diet plan.

The first type of food that you should try to avoid is trans fats. These will be found in a ton of your favorite foods such as pancakes, frosting, cake mixes, shortening, margarine, and French fries. Think of all your regular comfort foods and then know that most of these are not going to be allowed if you would like to prevent inflammation.

According to a study that was published in "The American Journal of Clinical Nutrition" in 2004, the relationship between inflammation and the intake of trans fats in women were looked at. The study would track the inflammation that was occurring in the participants by using monitors to find the levels of inflammation markets in the blood. This study found that the women who were consuming the largest amounts of trans fats were the ones that also had higher inflammation marker levels. So try to avoid these foods as much as possible if you are following one of these types of diet plans.

Next, you will need to make sure and avoid the saturated fats as well since these are not any better for you than the trans fats. Saturated fats are basically the ones that are found in animals such as meat, ice cream, pizza, and cheeseburgers. Red meat and dairy products that are full fat will have the most of these fats compared to any other product on the market.

According to the American Heart Association, these kinds of fats are known to stimulate inflammation inside the fat tissue. This will lead to insulin resistance in some people which is the start of type 2 diabetes and metabolic syndrome. Try to limit your intake of products with this fat in them in order to avoid more issues with inflammation.

While some grains are allowed on this diet plan, it is important to know the difference between those and the ones that you should stay away from. According to a study that was in "The Journal of Nutrition" in 2010 that examined the relationships between inflammation, refined grains, and whole grains, those who consumed whole grains would get less inflammation while those who were consuming the refined grains would have higher levels. When the grains have gone through refinement, many of the good nutrients that are inside them will be destroyed through the process. It is much better to choose whole grains and whole wheat options whenever possible. Then you are getting more of the good stuff in your diet and avoiding the extra sugars that are put in to the refined versions as well as the extra issues with inflammation.

Sugar is a big no while on an anti-inflammatory diet. This would include any sugary drinks or sodas that you might be used to having. A study that was published in "The American

Journal of Clinical Nutrition" took the time to investigate what effects sugary drinks would have on inflammation in normal men.

This diet chose to just look at moderate consumption of the drink to see how it would affect those who only had the sugar on occasion. The subjects who were in this study were told to consume 40 grams of a sugar beverage every day of the experiment. During this time, each of them experienced that their inflammation levels increased. In a regular bottle of pop there are 65 grams of sugar, a higher number than what is shown in this study so the results would be even more dramatic.

If you want to avoid the issues with your inflammation, you are going to have to cut sugar down as much as possible.

Chapter 14: Where To Find Recipes?

If you have decided to start the Mediterranean diet, one of the questions that you might be asking is where you can find recipes that will fit with this diet plan. It can be difficult to think of new and exciting recipes to try out with your family.

One way that you can incorporate new healthy meals into your diet is to find new recipes that you have never tried before. There are many places that you can look when you are looking for this diet plan. Some of these include looking online, looking on discussion boards, finding recipe books specifically for the Mediterranean diet, regular recipe books, and getting ideas from friends and family.

One place that you can look for ideas for recipes to try out with the anti-inflammatory diet is online. All you have to do is type in a couple of keywords and you will get hundreds of pages with tips and recipes for this diet plan. These websites will also show you how to prepare the meal and give you some options for side dishes and desserts to go with the meal. While you are online, you can also find answers to any questions that you might have about this diet.

Another place that you can look for recipes for this diet is on discussion boards. Discussion boards are full of people who have tried the different anti-inflammatory diets and have ideas on how to stay on the diet, how to keep motivated, different exercise plans, and recipes that you can try out. You can search either through a discussion board that is specifically for this diet or you can choose one that is just for a low-fat diet. If you find a discussion board that is not specifically for this diet it is important to remember that you might have to change some of the recipes in order for them to stick with this diet plan.

There are many recipe books for anti-inflammatory Diet that you can use in order to find something new to try for lunch or supper. The nice thing about a recipe book that is specific to this diet is that you do not need to modify the recipes at all. You will be able to choose any of the recipes that are in the book and know that they have already been pre-approved for this diet.

There is also the option just to look through a regular recipe book that you have at home or borrowed from a friend. You will have to go through each recipe that you are interested in and determine which ones will fit with this diet. You might be able to modify some of the recipes to make them fit with your diet. It is a good idea to pick recipes that include many fruits and vegetables and stay away from any recipe that uses red meat.

Friends and family are great resources to use in order to find recipes for this diet plan. If you know someone who is also on this diet, it is a good idea to ask them if they have any new recipes that they have tried that you might like. You could set up a fun night where you and a couple of friends get together and swap recipes. You will all leave and have many new recipes to try out when you get home.

You can also ask people in your family for recipes to try out. Even if they are not following this diet they might have some great recipes that will give you something new to try. You might have to modify a couple of them, but it is still nice to try new things every once in a while.

It does not matter too much where you find the recipes as long as they provide you with meals that you are going to enjoy and help prevent you from getting bored on this diet plan. There are a lot of different possibilities that you can find in a variety of places that will provide you with the meals that you need. You might want to take it slow in the beginning until you learn a little bit more about the diet plan and understand all of the rules that you will need to follow to be successful.

Once you have been on the diet plan a little while, you will be better equipped to eat right on this diet and can look all over the place to find the meals that you need.

PART 2 - Gluten

Chapter 15: Gluten Sensitivity vs. Celiac Disease

One common type of autoimmune disease is known as celiac disease. This disease causes the body to be intolerant to gluten, an ingredient found in bread, pasta, pastries, soup bases, etc. Why focus on celiac disease? Since celiac disease causes you to become intolerant to gluten, the cure is to eat a gluten-free diet.

Although celiac disease is focused on a gluten-free diet, other autoimmune diseases can be relieved with a gluten-free diet as well, such as Sjogren's syndrome and multiple sclerosis. Autoimmune diseases really can be healed by simply changing the way you eat!

There's a very fine line when it comes to simply being gluten intolerant or sensitive and having celiac disease. Celiac disease is an actual autoimmune disease, often occurring in conduction with other autoimmune diseases. People who have been diagnosed with celiac have a higher risk of having other autoimmune diseases. Your doctor can do a blood test to test for celiac. However, a biopsy via an endoscope is often required to confirm the diagnosis.

Should You Be Tested?

Although it may sound intimidating to get tested for celiac disease, you owe it to yourself to know about your body and how to keep up your health and well being. Autoimmune diseases can develop in anyone, but those with a higher risk or further indications of gluten intolerance include:

- Those with iron deficiency;
- People who have a family history of autoimmune diseases;
- People with osteoporosis development at a young age;
- People who have certain ethnic backgrounds. Hispanics and African Americans have a higher risk of developing the autoimmune disease, Lupus;
- Women with infertility;
- People who have Irritable Bowel Syndrome;
- People with liver disease.

Even if you're not one of these people, it's still a good idea to check with your doctor to see if you may develop or may already have celiac disease. The sooner you know, the sooner you can improve your diet and the symptoms that come with having celiac disease. In some cases, symptoms you think are ones of autoimmune diseases can just be symptoms of gluten intolerance or sensitivity.

What Is Gluten?

Gluten is a type of protein found in grain-based foods, such as bread, that holds the ingredients together. Think of it as glue that holds the components of bread or cakes together; it's what makes breads, cookies and other baked goods chewy.

For gluten intolerant people or those who have been diagnosed with celiac, gluten intake can cause inflammation in the small intestines. This prevents the body from absorbing the necessary nutrients that it needs to function properly. Those with celiac are required to go on a gluten-free diet due to the severe symptoms they experience, but that doesn't mean you can't go on a gluten-free diet or reduce your gluten intake.

Even though gluten comes mostly from grain-based foods, such as whole grain cereal and breads, it doesn't mean that you'll miss out on important nutrients like carbohydrates and fiber. There are other foods that can replace grains, such as fruits and vegetables.

Signs of Gluten Intolerance
You may be surprised to learn that gluten sensitivity doesn't always cause gastrointestinal symptoms. Here is a list of some of the symptoms of gluten sensitivity:

- Digestive/gastrointestinal problems such as bloating, gas, diarrhea and constipation;
- Migraines and headaches;
- Irrational mood swings;
- Fatigue after almost every meal that contains gluten;
- Chronic fatigue;
- Swelling in joints or joint pain;
- Skin rashes;
- Muscle aches;
- Acid reflux;

- Anemia;
- Irritability;
- Irregular weight loss or weight gain;
- Fibromyalgia
- Simply having an autoimmune diagnosis increases your chances of being intolerant

If you think you suffer from gluten sensitivity, keep a food journal for a week or even two, and write down a detailed list of your meals. Make a note of how you feel after your meals, and see if you notice symptoms related to your meals. For instance, you may repeatedly have increased joint pain the day after you eat pizza or have a large plate of pasta.

Remember, just because you test negative for celiac doesn't mean you aren't gluten intolerant. We don't have a test available yet that can accurately test for sensitivity. The best test is your own body!

Chapter 16: Living Gluten-Free

Living a gluten-free lifestyle is an option for everyone. When you decide to have a gluten-free diet, it also means that you're committed to having a gluten-free lifestyle. It's not a fad diet, either. It's a lifestyle change to becoming a healthier person and living a more comfortable life with any autoimmune disease or sensitivity your body has developed.

Benefits of Going Gluten-Free
Going gluten-free is nothing less than rewarding and healing for the body, whether you have an autoimmune disease or gluten sensitivity. Some of the benefits include:

- Saying goodbye to stomach aches and pains! Gluten in food causes the intestines to react negatively to it, causing inflammation and irritation. Having a gluten-free diet will help ease those stomach pains and heal any damage that may have been caused to the intestines. Since the intestines may be damaged, your body will have a harder time absorbing nutrients. It will be thanking you for the additional nutrients!

- Decrease fatigue. Removing gluten reduces inflammation in the body allowing you to have more energy. When your body is no longer having a reaction to gluten, and the immune system is no longer activated by it, there is decreased inflammation and increased energy.

- Going gluten-free will help stabilize your insulin levels. Foods that contain wheat or other gluten ingredients cause your insulin levels to rise and drop very quickly, which can affect your energy levels. Going gluten-free will help relieve you from unstable insulin levels.

- There are more gluten-free products out in the market. More companies are making it easier to find gluten-free foods and making it easier for you to go on a gluten-free diet. This awareness is spreading, and more people are going gluten-free to improve their health.

- Having a gluten-free lifestyle encourages you to be more aware of what you eat. You're aiming to become healthier and ease any aches and pains you have from an autoimmune disease or gluten sensitivity. You'll now be checking food labels and becoming more health conscious.

Going gluten-free isn't a fad: it's what can heal you from an autoimmune disease and help you live a more comfortable, pain free lifestyle. Consider these benefits, knowing a simple change in eating habits can save you from years of suffering.

Why Eat A Gluten Free Diet?

Some individuals have no choice but to follow a gluten free lifestyle due to the way their bodies process it. Celiac disease is a type of autoimmune disorder that results in the body rejecting gluten instead of processing it. The gluten is seen as a toxin to their bodies and it can create very serious health problems.

The severity of the reaction can vary based on the individual and the amount of gluten that they consume. A gluten allergy is extremely common, but it is very rarely diagnosed. Today, more people are informed about the symptoms and more medical professionals are testing for it.

This is why the number of children with sensitivity to gluten is being identified. There are adults that have struggled with their health for their entire life though because this gluten problem was never addressed. The sooner that a person is diagnosed though the sooner changes to their diet can be implemented.

It is believed that 1 in 133 people have some form of Celiac disease. The problem is that when they are consuming gluten their small intestine is being damaged. This creates problems with the small intestine successfully absorbing nutrients that the body needs. Some reports indicate approximately 83% of the cases though aren't diagnosed.

Celiac disease is genetic so if anyone in your family has it then your risk increases. Some individuals have several symptoms and others don't have any at all. There are more than 300 possible symptoms that can occur, but these are the most common:

- Abdominal pain
- Anemia
- Bloating
- Bone pain
- Chronic fatigue
- Depression
- Diarrhea
- Fertility problems
- Gas
- Headaches
- Weight changes

Children may have some other symptoms that develop including:
- Behavioral changes
- Dental enamel damage
- Distended abdomen
- Failure to gain weight or height at their percentile

In order to confirm such a diagnosis, blood work is completed. If it comes back positive, than a biopsy of the small intestine will be done to see if the lining has been damaged as well as the degree of any damage that has occurred. There is no cure for Celiac disease other than to follow a gluten free diet.

Doing so allow the small intestine to heal and in time it can allow a person to make a full recovery. Their body will start being able to use the nutrients that they consume for better overall health. The problem will get worse if dietary changes aren't made including malnutrition, osteoporosis, neurological problems, and Lymphoma.

Request testing for you and your children if possible because so many people go undiagnosed with this type of problem. If you think this could be the issue, don't want until your doctor brings up the idea of the testing. Ask your family members too in order to determine if there is a high chance of it occurring for you or your child.

Some individuals develop Dermatitis Herpetiformis, often referred to as DH, which is a type of Celiac disease that affects the skin. In order to diagnosis it blood work and a skin biopsy are conducted. The only cure for it is also a gluten free diet.

Such a test is a good idea as this type of skin problem is often mistaken for Eczema. It can be very frustrating when the medication for Eczema is given but the condition either stays the same or gets worse. Until the diet is changed then the skin isn't going to clear up.

Many people make the choice to have a gluten free diet even though they don't have the disease. Some have a family history of many health problems and they are being as proactive as possible to reduce the risk of serious health concerns for them personally.

If you decide to make this your lifestyle due to your own personal beliefs, you need to stand up for it. Don't let others that don't agree with you or that don't understand your decision to create problems or doubts for you. Not everyone in your life will be supportive about it but the majority of people will.

A gluten free lifestyle isn't something to be shy about, to be ashamed of, or that you need to hide. It may be different from other people and the food choices they make but that is okay. It is about doing what is right for you and for your family in this regard so don't succumb to peer pressure.

Parents try to do all they can to create a world for their children that is fair, that is fun, and that is rewarding. Yet there can be issues with children that society as a whole isn't kind about. For example, children that have ADD or ADHD or those with Autism.

As the parent of a child with those types of issues, it can be exhausting. It can be hard for you and your partner to deal with on a daily basis. You may feel like you have been isolated by your friends and family because of it. Not giving up on your child though is important.

Some parents have found that their child did significantly improve by removing gluten from their diet. This was a better option or them than medicating their child. When there are behavior issues that aren't explained, it is definitely worth trying a gluten free diet for a few months and monitoring the behavior of your child.

If you see improvements, then that is encouraging and you should continue the diet. It could make a huge difference in the happiness of your child, in the dynamics of your household, and even how your child is accepted socially.

There are a few studies out there that indicate a gluten free diet can be a way to reduce symptoms of other forms of autoimmune deficiencies too. This includes:
- Cystic Fibrosis
- Multiple Sclerosis
- Thyroid Disease

Such information is very encouraging because it can be very upsetting to deal with the symptoms of these autoimmune deficiencies. They can create pain, fatigue, and other symptoms that affect every element of a person's life. If changing to a gluten free diet can make these health problems more manageable, isn't it worth it to consider?

Other individuals have taken on a gluten free lifestyle due to having a child or partner that needs to follow such a diet plan. It is certainly easier to create meals that everyone in the household can consume rather than making something different from the person that can't have gluten. Plus, if a parent has a gluten related issue that it is very possible children in the household will at some point. Teaching them a healthier way of eating from an early age is important.

There are people that choose not to consume gluten because they feel better removing it from their diet. While they didn't test positive for Celiac disease, they may have some sort of wheat allergy. They may have an intolerance or sensitivity to gluten.

They often have gas or bloating when they consume it so they have removed if from their diet to be more comfortable. They don't have damage to the small intestine due to the gluten but they just feel better overall by not consuming it anymore. No one wants to try to get through their day continually with bloating and gas. It can make it hard to focus on work, social activities, and even intimate relationships. With the anxiety gone about such symptoms, it can give a person a refreshing and upbeat outlook about life that was missing before.

Weight loss and weight maintenance has also been a reason to stop consuming gluten. The craving for sweets can make it hard to stick to a good diet plan but many people find they don't have cravings after a few weeks of a gluten free diet.

They also find that they lose weight and keep it off because they are no longer reaching for foods that have empty calories or snacks that are processed. Such changes can also do wonders for the amount of energy a person has.

Many people feel that they have been on a losing course for weight loss for quite some time. They don't have the willpower to stick with a program that is restricting them and they really shouldn't. Fad diets may be very popular but they are really just setting people up to fail. Many people find that they can stick with a gluten free diet and that they do lose weight.

There are a few reasons for that to occur. As previously mentioned, the cravings go away and that makes selecting healthier choices easier. Reducing the amount of processed foods that are consumed means that there is less harmful carbs that the body will store as fat. There is also less sugar intake that will be stored as fat.

The increased energy with this lifestyle also gives someone that help them may need to really exercise. They may have had a hard time doing so before but now they have both the energy and the motivation to stick with a plan of action. As they feel better and their mood improves it becomes a path that they would like to continue going down.

The verdict is still out there by the experts though regarding recommending the gluten free diet for weight loss. Since it can't be proven without in depth and time consuming studies you won't find doctor's that readily recommend it. However, you will find plenty of people that state it was the change that allowed them to feel great and to drop the pounds when nothing else worked.

If you have hit a point where you feel like losing weight is a lost cause, you may wish to give this type of lifestyle a try for a 90 day period. If you find that you feel better, you have more energy, and that you have lost weight then it is an option to continue with it.

Regardless of your reason for deciding to follow a gluten free diet – by necessity or by choice – it doesn't have to be hard and it doesn't have to be time consuming. It doesn't mean that you have a huge grocery bill or that you can't enjoy going out to eat.

If you travel often, you may be worried but you can use the internet to help you find great menu choices and restaurants anywhere you may go that offer gluten free selections. You have the ability to make this work for you and all of the information you need is at your fingertips!

Children and Gluten Free Diets

If your child is following a gluten free diet – by necessity or by your parenting choice – talk to them about it. It is amazing what children can learn even from an early age about making good food choices. Explain to them the importance of their food choices.

Let them know that if they are in doubt about what they can eat then they should refrain from consuming it until they get approval from an adult. Make sure your child's gluten diet is well known when they go to stay with a friend too. You can talk to the parent's in advance to make accommodations.

Offer to send a gluten free meal and snacks so that they don't feel obligated to buy special items for your child to be a guest in their home. This also reduces the risk that they may not properly follow labeling due to not having enough information to make the right choices.

At the other end of that spectrum, think about elderly individuals you may be responsible for. If you make their meals or they are in an assisted care facility they may need a gluten free diet plan. Make sure anyone that is in charge of their care understands what they can eat and what they can't.

Exercise

It is very important to point out that daily exercise is important for people of all ages. Taking part in a gluten free diet is a step in the right direction for overall health, losing weight, and maintaining a healthy body weight. Exercise still needs to be a part of the daily routine. Many individuals didn't exercise enough before due to their diet.

They continually felt fatigued and sluggish so it was hard for them to take part in working out. Once they changed to a gluten free diet though they found that they were able to benefit from the additional energy. They were energetic all day long too without peaks and valleys in there that once required a sugar intake as a pick me up.

Talk to your doctor about starting any new exercise program. Keep in mind that if you make too many changes at once to your lifestyle it will be hard to stick with it. Focus on the dietary changes and becoming familiar with what you can eat and what you can't first.

Then as your energy level increases and you are getting comfortable with your dietary changes you can look at the exercise plan. Find forms of exercise you can take part in that are at your fitness level. You should also take part in forms of exercise that you will enjoy so you will stick with them.

Chapter 17: How to Get Started on a Gluten-Free Diet

To help you get started on a gluten-free diet, read these effective tips:

- Start slow. Get the basics of a gluten-free diet under your belt first before you include more foods into your diet. You should take your gluten-free lifestyle education slow as well; it can be overwhelming when you start a new diet and lifestyle, so learn as you go. For now, learn the basics first and get those down before you move on to the next stage of a gluten-free lifestyle. You can start with your gluten-free diet, and then move on to gluten-proof the rest of your environment, from your kitchen to your bathroom. Yes, gluten can be found in many products, not just food.

- Talk to a professional nutritionist or dietitian who specializes in gluten-free diets. What better way to start a gluten-free diet than to talk to a professional.

You can also search for blogs or websites created by certified nutritionists who are adept to gluten-free eating and lifestyles. Although you may be hesitant about this tip, it's always best to consult a professional to see if they can come up with a specific, gluten-free eating plan for you.

- Learn how to read food labels. When it comes to living a gluten-free lifestyle, it does take practice and learning. It is a lifestyle change, and it'll take at least a couple of weeks for you to learn the ropes of a gluten-free diet. However, once you learn the brands that are safe for you to purchase, you'll quickly be on your way to feeling better, fast.

- Watch for hidden gluten. One type of label food used by many companies is "wheat-free", which is not the same as gluten free. Always check the food labels to confirm that something is gluten-free. Gluten can also be hidden under other words. Watch out for words like spelt, hydrolyzed wheat protein, bulgar, durum and malt, or barley malt. All of these are gluten hidden under different names.

- Clean out your cupboards and pantry. Say goodbye to gluten foods in your kitchen! Take the time to toss out any food that contains gluten in it so you're not tempted to eat it. If you have housemates, it can be helpful at first to label products that are gluten free until you learn which brands are safe to eat. Even your kitchen tools may need to be gluten-proof to help you stick to your gluten-free path. Porous kitchen utensils, such as wooden spoons, may harbor gluten in its pores, cracks, creases, etc., so it's important to keep your kitchen utensils clean or get new ones.

- Make a list of what you can't eat on a gluten-free diet and keep it in your kitchen at all times. Make it easier on yourself and know what types of foods you can't eat on a gluten-free diet by doing this exercise. You'll always know what to stay away from when you have a list nearby.

- Try exotic fruits and vegetables. Bok choy and star fruits are examples of exotic produce you can try. When you go gluten-free, fruits and veggies will always be available for you to try, so get into a curious, adventurous mindset and try out different produce so that you don't get bored with food.

- Find gluten-free recipes on websites or blogs. Even though the gluten-free lifestyle may seem restrictive, there are countless ways for you to enjoy gluten-free food. There are many people who are willing to help others living a gluten-free lifestyle, so find blogs and sites that share gluten-free recipes. Going gluten-free doesn't mean you need to make this complicated or have to make food that's not appetizing. You're just making a positive lifestyle change to improve your health and illness.

- Try out the Paleo diet. The Paleo diet, also known as the Caveman diet, doesn't include any grains, such as cereals, breads, etc. This means that you'll be able to follow an easy, healthy eating program that is also gluten-free.

Take pride in your gluten-free lifestyle. Whether you have the option to go gluten-free or you've been diagnosed with Celiac disease and are forced to go gluten-free, take pride in it! You're doing this to become a healthier person, and there's no shame in that. Think about it this way: the foods you eat have gluten in them are only hurting you. Do you want to harm yourself for short term pleasure or relieve yourself from inflammation and pain?

Chapter 18 - Quick Start Guide - What You Can and Can't Eat

First, you should know about the types of foods and ingredients you should stay away from when on a gluten-free diet. Here is a list of the most common foods that you can't eat when you go gluten-free:

- Breaded meat e.g., fried chicken
- rye
- Barley
- Flour made from barley, rye or wheat
- Wheat germ
- Wheat
- Kamut
- Malted milk
- Matzo
- Bran/Oat
- Spelt
- Triticale (cross between wheat and rye)
- Couscous

But don't worry – even though you'll have to watch what you eat more closely, there are way more foods that you can eat. Some examples are:

- All fruits
- All vegetables
- Fresh meats and seafood that hasn't been marinaded, breaded or coated with batter
- Beans
- Nuts and seeds
- Flax
- Arrowroot
- Rice
- Corn (including popcorn and tortillas)
- Quinoa
- Tapioca
- Millet
- Potato flour and other gluten-free flours

Don't think of going on a gluten-free diet as restrictive. Many people have a fear of not being allowed to do something or eat something, so they get scared to try a new diet. It's true that going gluten-free means eating food that doesn't have gluten in it, that doesn't mean you'll have boring, tasteless meals. There are many ways for you to flavor your foods and make it delicious.

Another thing to be warned about when you're going gluten-free: there are hidden gluten ingredients in food products. These ingredients can be camouflaged under a different name. Even though some people won't be affected by a small amount of gluten, it's still important to know the hidden gluten ingredients found in food products. Some food products that contain hidden gluten include:

- Canned soups and broth
- Bottled salad dressings
- Chips and crackers
- Bottled sauces
- Soy sauce
- Beer
- Brown rice syrup
- Imitation crab meat
- Vanilla extract

All of the products mentioned above are now sold in gluten free versions. However, always check the food label to make sure you're buying the correct product.

Chapter 19: How to Manage Your Gluten-Free Lifestyle

It's a new lifestyle, so of course you're going to have slip-ups and hard times here and there, but that's okay. You can still manage your life easily when you make the switch to gluten-free. Also, this section is not just about managing your gluten-free lifestyle, but also the autoimmune disease you've been diagnosed with, if applicable.

Here are a few tips to get you through:

- Plan out your meals each week. Take a day to plan out your meals and go grocery shopping so that you're prepared. If you do all of your shopping sporadically or cook last minute, you can end up rushing the process and not enjoy your gluten-free foods.

- Check on Amazon before you go grocery shopping. Is there a gluten-free product you'd like to buy but it pushes you outside your grocery budget? Check Amazon or other internet sources for lower prices.

Check your local yellow pages or do an internet search for your city and find gluten free shops. Many cities have entire stores dedicated to gluten free foods. It can take a little longer at first, but it's worth getting high-quality, gluten-free items so that you can have fantastic meals all the time. Before you know it, you'll be an expert!

- Dine out without fear. Even when you go out to eat, you don't need to slip up on your gluten-free diet and risk your health. Many restaurants now have gluten free menus. Check the internet before you dine out to see the menu or obtain the ingredient list if it's a restaurant you are unsure of. It may sound tedious, but you can always talk to your server and ask questions about the dish you're interested in.

- Join a gluten-free community. Sometimes, it's going to be hard to keep up with your gluten-free diet and all the things you need to learn about living a gluten-free lifestyle. Finding a gluten-free community online or in your local area can help give you added support, knowledge, and encouragement. Find out if the community has a forum or monthly meetings you can participate in or any type of event you can join. Make going gluten-free a fun experience for yourself, and connect with others who are going through the same things you are.

- Reach out to family members and friends about your new lifestyle change. Be assertive about your lifestyle change and commitment to it by talking to close family members and friends about it. Whenever they invite you over for a meal or another event that includes food, talk to them about the certain foods you can't eat. Many people are more than happy to ensure that you, as their guest, will be comfortable and enjoy being at their home. You can always offer to bring your own food or bread, for instance, in order to make them feel more comfortable in what they are serving.

- Prepare meals ahead of time. No matter what lifestyle you lead, this is one of the most classic tips of all time when it comes to managing your diet. Preparing your meals ahead of time will help you avoid the temptation to go back to your old eating habits. Pick a day of the week to prepare all your meals and separate them into small bowls or containers. Label them for each meal and each day of the week.

- Find helpful smartphone apps. There are many smartphone apps that can help you manage your gluten-free lifestyle. Most of these apps will help you eat better and dine out in a gluten-free fashion.

- Make a budget. There are many food options out there that require you to dig deep in your wallet for extra money to buy it, but gluten-free doesn't have to be expensive. Take the time to figure out your budget along with the costs of the food products you plan to buy. You can check prices on your grocery store's website or take some time to investigate the product prices at the store.

How to Plan a Gluten-Free Diet

Meal planning is essential for any diet. Since you're making a lifestyle change, you want to make sure you have the right meal plans in place so that you get all essential nutrients.

Grocery Shopping

Planning your meals is an important part of a gluten free lifestyle. It reduces the need for you to make an unhealthy choice because you are pushed for time. Plan your snacks too so that you always have something you can reach for when you get hungry. You don't have to be overwhelmed by the task of going to the grocery store though.

There are more stores that offer gluten free products than you may realize. The demand for them as well as the variety of options continues to grow all the time. You can go online to find out where to shop locally for those items you want. If you aren't finding enough selection, talk to the manager.

They may be willing to add a few gluten free items to what they normally stock if customers ask for it. Studies show that as of 2012, approximately 15% of customers were shopping for only gluten free products. Up to 25% were buying products gluten free as they have scaled down on the volume of gluten that they consume.

The predictions from U.S. News and World Report is that this percentage is only going to continue to climb in the future. Retailers that sell groceries are certainly going to be paying attention to this information as well and preparing the shelves in their stores to meet that demand.

Being well informed is important when you are shopping for gluten free products. Some of the common foods you may normally reach for to add to your basket contain gluten including:

- Bagels
- Cereal
- Crackers
- Pasta
- Pizza

Identifying what you can safely eat and what you can't is important so that you can be a great shopper. To help you feel better about all of this, focus on what you can eat and not what you are giving up.

Remember the many health benefits that you will gain when you start to feel your willpower slipping. The more you shop for gluten free items, the easier it becomes. Soon, it will be second nature for you when you enter the store.

Read Labels Carefully!

Different brands of products can contain gluten or not so you need to become familiar with the products out there. Don't be in a rush when you shop so that you can take all the time you need to read labels. Some products say gluten free and others say low gluten.

Fruits and Vegetables

Any fresh fruits and fresh vegetables that you see in the grocery store aren't processed and they are gluten free. You can buy sweet potatoes and white potatoes as they don't contain any gluten either. Both dry beans and peas are acceptable.

Dairy

Just about all of the milk and cheese that you will find at the grocery store are free of gluten. There are some exceptions though so you need to carefully read labels. Some processed cheese products have wheat in them and blue cheese does. If you buy plain yogurt there is no gluten. However, if you buy various flavors then there can be so always check the labels.

Meat, Fish, Pork, & Poultry

Look for lean cuts of meat, pork, and poultry. Only buy fresh fish and other forms of seafood. When you are looking at canned or frozen products in this category, many of them can contain gluten due to the processing. Always take the time to carefully read the labels. When possible, use fresh products instead of frozen or canned as they are better for you.

Grains

Select grains that are free of gluten. You will find that you can pick the varieties you like too. There are gluten free options with white, brown, and wild rice so your choice won't be limited.

Shopping List

A typical gluten-free grocery list:

- Beans (any kind)
- Buckwheat
- Butter
- Unprocessed cheese
- Cornmeal, grits, masa and/or polenta
- Eggs

- Flax seeds
- Vegetable, canola or olive oil
- Gluten-free oats / oatmeal
- Milk
- Sweet and baking potatoes
- Gluten-free yogurt
- All fresh vegetables and fruits
- Tofu
- Tamari
- Nuts and seeds

The foods on this shopping list are gluten-free. You want to make sure you include nutritious foods on your shopping list so that you get well-rounded meals. Here are a few more tips on planning your meals and ensuring you continue to eat healthy:

- Eat vegetables at every meal, if possible. If you're making an omelet for breakfast, add cubed tomatoes and spinach leaves to give it a health kick. For lunch, you can have a leafy, green salad with homemade, gluten-free salad dressing. For dinner, add steamed vegetables tossed in garlic butter with your main dish. Vegetables are always gluten-free, so make sure that you get enough servings of it during the day to keep you full. Also, eat a variety of vegetables so that you get more essential nutrients in your body.

- Watch out for excess sugar and fat. Sometimes, products that are labeled gluten-free can have additional sugar and fat to make the food taste better. Make sure to check the labels so you don't have too much sugar going into your system. The excess sugar can cause more health problems for you down the road.

- Plan your meals around natural, gluten-free foods. Meals don't have to be complicated, and you can get your own ideas for recipes with gluten-free ingredients. Take these meals for example:

  ○ Scrambled eggs with gluten-free, unprocessed cheese and bacon with a side bowl of fresh fruit
  ○ Baked potato loaded with bacon bits, cheese, sour cream, green onion and steamed vegetables
  ○ Bean, cheese and grilled chicken burritos made with corn tortillas instead of flour tortillas
  ○ Baked or grilled fish with steamed vegetables
  ○ Corn tortilla chips with cheese, seasoned beef and salsa

- Learn to make gluten-free, homemade food. Just because you can't eating gluten doesn't mean you have to swear off bread or other foods you love. There are still ways for you to create healthy, gluten-free versions of your favorites; all you need to do is figure out the gluten type ingredients used in them and substitute it with gluten-free ingredients. You can also make gluten-free sauces and salad dressings at home and freeze them until ready to use.

Dining Out

When it comes to dining out, spend some time looking online to identify which restaurants offer you such dishes. This is very important if you are traveling and aren't familiar with the area. With the technology today, you can use your smartphone or a laptop to see what is available where you happen to be.

If you aren't able to do that, ask when you arrive about any gluten free foods that they may offer. Some locations are willing to make something special for you. With more restaurants trying to appease the needs of everyone it is possible they will work with you. Try to arrive at off peak times so they can provide you with personalized service.

There are some common items you can get though that would be fine. For example, order chicken or fish with a side of vegetables. You can also get a baked potato and a salad. You may want to ask what type of oil that fish or chicken is cooked in though as some of them do contain gluten.

There is a great deal of gluten in various marinades and sauces. If you aren't sure they are free of gluten it is best to avoid them. You can ask for them to be put on the side and most restaurants will be happy to comply. Don't expect there to be gluten free bread or crackers though so make sure you don't reach for them unless you are positive!

It is fine to consume champagne and wine as they are made from grapes. However, most beer is going to be off limits due to the grains they use to make them. You will find some gluten free beer offers though in many restaurants so it doesn't hurt to ask. You can also consider various forms of mixed drinks.

If dessert is something you just don't want to pass up, you aren't going to have to. There are some great choices in this category too. If the restaurant is gluten free friendly they may have flourless cake available. You can also consider sorbet, sherbet, fresh fruit, or ice cream. They are universal options so there is a very good chance they will be available.

Some labels on products aren't as clear as they should be when it comes to determining if they contain gluten or not. If that is the case with a particular product, err on the side of caution. Don't buy it and you can do some research at home about it. You can always buy that product on your next shopping trip if you do find it is actually free of gluten.

The more you are aware of what you can eat and what you shouldn't, the easier it is for you to shop and for your to dine out without stress or worry. See appendix 1 for a list to help you as you work to become more familiar with your options.

Recipes

It is a good idea to add the following items to your shopping list and to keep them on hand in your kitchen. They are commonly called for in gluten free recipes. You can also use them when you run low on food items for your menu to make something.

- Gluten free baking mix
- Gluten free crackers
- Gluten free bread crumbs
- Gluten free flour
- Gluten free snacks
- Guar Gum
- Quinoa
- Rice (brown or white depending on your preference)
- Xantham Gum

With these items you can also use some of your favorite recipes but with a gluten free value to them. It can be both fun and productive to get creative with those recipes. Here are some great tips for starting with such replacements:

- Binders – Use Xanthan Gum, Guar Gum, or gelatin.
- Breading – Wheat or gluten free bread crumbs or crushed potato chips.
- Flour – Use gluten free flour mix or cornstarch. There are plenty of options to consider including amaranth and sorghum.
- Thickening – Use cornstarch or gluten free baking mix. For a sweet recipe, use dry pudding mix.

The internet is a wonderful resource for finding various gluten free recipes to try. You will enjoy the new tastes and you will gain more confidence in this lifestyle choice as you are able to create meals you and your family love. You can also buy gluten free cookbooks, magazines, or exchange recipes with others that are also eating gluten free.

Here are some great ideas to get you started. Try some new recipes and create a file for those that you really like. As your file grows you can ensure lots of variety in your diet so you don't feel restricted or bored by eating the same thing over and over again.

Meal Ideas
Breakfast
Yogurt is a great option but make sure it is gluten free as many varieties aren't. Both Stonyfield and Chobani are certified by the Gluten Intolerant Group. You can use the yogurt as a basis for a delicious tasting smoothie too.

There are various brands of gluten free cereal by General Mills and Nature's Path. If you like hot cereal consider Cream of Buckwheat. There are also oats that are certified to be gluten free. Eggs that are fried or scrambled are a great way to start the day due to the amount of protein they offer.

Lunch

Lunch meat is a great choice for a convenient and gluten free option, but make sure it isn't processed. A salad can be a choice that works for you due to all of the vegetables. You have to be careful though as some of the cheese items and various dressings can have gluten in them.

Nachos consisting of tortilla chips and some melted cheese that is gluten free is a change from your basic lunch and very appetizing. Peanut butter on gluten free bread is another great consideration.

Dinner

Lean cuts of meat including beef, pork, and poultry are great choices. You can also consume fresh fish or other seafood. Adding fresh vegetables and your choice of potatoes offers you a wonderful meal without gluten in no time at all. You can also replace the potatoes with your choice of gluten free rice.

Snacks

Gluten free snacks you can enjoy between meals will keep you on track. Cut up fresh fruit and vegetables so you can grab them and go. You can pack them to take in the car or to have at your desk while working.

There are plenty of types of cheese that don't contain gluten, and they are wonderful for snacking. They also help you to get your calcium. With certain flavors of cheese you need to be careful as they can have some gluten in them so always read the packaging. Kids seem to really enjoy those individually wrapped cheese sticks.

While you should only consume chips in moderation, they are also gluten free when it comes to many varieties including most of those offered by Frito Lay. For a lower calorie snack consider popcorn. Make some hardboiled eggs and consume them when you need a snack. They will give you lots of energy.

Desserts
Both children and adults enjoy dessert, and you don't have to eliminate it due to a gluten free diet. Various brands of pudding are free of gluten and you will have a variety of flavors to pick from. Ice cream can also be a wonderful treat but you need to pay attention to the labels. So many ice cream varieties these days are packed with goodies so you need to pay attention to what is in there.

Cross Contamination
It is very important that you think about the risk of cross contamination in your own kitchen as well as those of others that prepare gluten free meals for you or your family. If the same tools are used to prepare such items as those that do have gluten then there can be some contamination.

Even a small amount of gluten can be dangerous to certain individuals so care has to be taken to prevent this. It is one more reason why changing the entire family to a gluten free diet may be the best option to consider.

Holidays
For many people, the holidays can be tough due to the restrictions of the diet. There can be parties to attend and

various events where you have to be very careful about what you eat.

You may decide to make dinner at your own home and offer a gluten free meal for all. It is certainly an option to consider. Prepare yourself for the holidays and have a few items you can take along for snacks with you in case an event isn't gluten free friendly.

Chapter 20: Supplements for a Gluten-Free Dieter

Now, let's go over the vitamins and supplements you may want to consider while on a gluten-free diet:

- Fiber – With breads, cereals, and oats (non gluten-free) out of the picture, fiber is needed in another source. You can get fiber from fruits, prunes, popcorn, and vegetables, but there are supplements you can take to get your fiber fill for the day.

- Folate – Often called folic acid. Folate is necessary for cell growth and development. It's also known to prevent birth defects, and since women who are in their child-bearing years may have to go on a gluten-free diet, they'll have to find other sources for folate since gluten-containing foods have more folate in them. Natural folate sources include spinach, peanuts, asparagus, broccoli and green peas. There are supplements for folic acid as well.

- Calcium – Some people who are sensitive to gluten or have Celiac disease, may suffer from premature osteoporosis or thinning bones. Calcium is needed to strengthen bones, so it's an important nutrient. You can drink milk on a gluten-free diet, but if you're also lactose intolerant, supplements may work better for you.

- Vitamin D – As the partner to calcium, vitamin D is necessary for absorbing calcium, so it's another essential nutrient. Since many people who have Celiac disease are shown to be deficient in calcium and vitamin D, taking supplements or eating/drinking fortified vitamin D foods, such as gluten-free yogurt, gluten-free orange juice and milk, can help them get the necessary vitamin D into their body.

- Iron – Many people who have autoimmune diseases, suffer from anemia. You can find iron in leafy, green vegetables and meat.

- Vitamin B12 – Vitamin B12 helps you fight fatigue, and many gluten containing foods have this vitamin. Since you're going gluten-free, there are other ways to obtain this vitamin and maintain your health. You can find vitamin B12 in meats, organ meats (e.g., liver), fish and milk.

Supplements can be found for each of these vitamins and minerals, but it's always better to eat natural foods to get your nutrients. You may have to eat more to get the daily nutrients that your body needs, but you can also vary the foods you eat to get those nutrients.

Changing a lifestyle and diet isn't easy, but at least give this new lifestyle a try. Make a commitment to try it for one month. Use a journal to track your progress, and, at the end of one month, see how much better you feel.

When to Expect Results

The main reason to go on a gluten-free diet is to ease any symptoms you're suffering from and to help heal yourself. Any drastic change in your diet and lifestyle will force your body to adjust to the change, so results can vary among people. You may notice improvements within a week and start to feel better and healthier. Sometimes, it may take up to a month or more to be completely free of your gluten sensitivity or intolerance symptoms. People with true Celiac disease sometimes require a whole year or more of gluten-free eating to completely heal the damage in the intestinal tract. However, if you stick to the diet you'll see results faster and feel better quicker.

Support

Your decision to be gluten free is one you should feel proud of no matter why you have made that decision. It is a good idea to get a support system in place as soon as you can about it. Share with your family, friends, and co-workers about your lifestyle change and what it entails. You will be pleasantly surprised at the many people that support you and even think about making the change for their own household.

Tell your healthcare providers about such changes too if they haven't mandated it due to a medical necessity. You will find that most medical professionals are very supportive of this type of dietary change.

Being well informed is important so you should consider magazines, books, and websites. However, you need to make sure you fully explore the credibility of such resources or you will end up with so much conflicting information it can make your head spin.

If you have questions, there are some very good organizations where you can direct your questions. They include the Celiac Disease Foundation and the Gluten Intolerance Group.

There are plenty of online forums where you can get support and meet new people. You may find it useful to be able to ask questions from those that are also going through similar changes in their lifestyle.

Being able to share recipes, to vent when you are discouraged, and even to be able to get some encouragement when you really need it is important. You can also offer support to others from time to time so it becomes a give and take.

Don't underestimate the value of this type of support as it helps to educate people about gluten free diets. The volume of the masses can also encourage more gluten free products in restaurants and grocery stores.

If you have children, make sure that their caregivers and teachers know they are on a gluten free diet. You may need to send your child with their lunch daily as the school or daycare lunch menu may not reflect this choice.

You may need to provide snacks too but if you feel this is the right method for your household then your caregiver and the school should work with you. Check to see if there are any gluten free cooking classes offered in your community.

This can be a great way to learn some new cooking methods, try some delicious recipes, and make some terrific friends that you can count on to help you as you help them get used to these dietary changes. You may find working with a dietician is useful as well.

Conclusion

Inflammation is body's response against any local or foreign invading organisms. The body uses this response in order to eliminate and fight against the foreign or local invaders. When any microorganism or any other irritants is entered the body, the body's immune system is activated, and tries to eliminate the invaders, minimize the injury and start the healing process at the injury site.

Inflammation is often associated with infection, but it is important to remember that most infections can cause inflammation, but not every inflammation means an infection. Inflammation is very important element of healing process, as without it, healing process cannot begin. However, sometimes inflammation can be caused by an autoimmune disease like rheumatoid arthritis, Addison's disease, etc.

Since there is more than one reason for inflammation, you should investigate all possibilities for the inflammation, not just the possibility of injury. Autoimmune diseases are typically diagnosed when other symptoms begin to manifest or the disorder decides to have a serious flare and appear as though it is another illness or injury.

Acute inflammation begins just after the injury and attempts to counteract the injury by eliminating the invaders and initiating the healing process. If acute inflammation fails to remove the causative agent from the injury site, then it leads to chronic inflammation that usually begins after some days of acute inflammation and can last for several months to years. There are some blood tests available for inflammation. During inflammation, several vascular and chemical changes are going on that cause swelling, itching, redness and pain at the affected area.

Poor eating habits, sedentary life style, too much stress, inadequate sleep and busy life schedules are high risk factors for inflammation. By adjusting lifestyle and diet habits, the symptoms of inflammation can be weakened. Some herbs and foods known to have anti-inflammatory effects and they can be beneficial in reducing and treating inflammatory disorders and inflammation. Some medications for the inflammation are available and can help in treating and managing the disorder.

I hope this book has given you the tools to start your journey on an anti inflammatory/ gluten-free diet. Inflammation caused from autoimmune diseases is exacerbated by gluten in the many people that are gluten sensitive.

Unfortunately, there isn't a test for gluten sensitivity; only a test for celiac disease. The best test is YOU! Your body tells you when it's sick and it will tell you when it's getting better. We'll never know until you go on a gluten-free diet. Don't you think you're worth it? I certainly do!

Appendix

You can consume any gluten free grain products including:

- Amaranth
- Buckwheat
- Corn flour
- Cornmeal
- Grits
- Millet
- Montina
- Quinoa
- Rice (brown, white, enriched, or basmati)
- Sorghum
- Soy
- Vegetable oil

Common Staples:

- Cheese (most blends but read the labels)
- Beans
- Butter
- Lean meats
- Legumes
- Fresh fruit
- Fresh seafood
- Fresh vegetables
- Margarine
- Milk
- Yogurt (plain, read the labels on flavored)

You May Enjoy Mary's Other Book On Autoimmune Disease Diets

Autoimmune Disease Inflammation Diet: Natural Pain Relief and Disease Control

hyperurl.co/autoimmune

RECOMMEDED READING

HEALING: Heal Your Mind, Heal Your Body: Change Your Life

hyperurl.co/selfhealing

SELF ESTEEM: Confidence Building: Overcome Fear, Stress and Anxiety: Self Help Guide

hyperurl.co/selfesteem

MEDICAL MARIJUANA and Pain Free Living

smarturl.it/mja

Anger: Natural Treatments To Manage Frustration And Stress

hyperurl.co/anger

References

http://www.heart.org/HEARTORG/Conditions/Inflammation-and-Heart-Disease_UCM_432150_Article.jsp#

http://www.thesurvivaldoctor.com/2013/02/23/inflammation-and-your-heart-treatment-explanation-and-advice/

http://www.patient.co.uk/health/Blood-Test-Detecting-Inflammation.htm

http://scdlifestyle.com/2012/10/chronic-inflammation-signs-symptoms-and-testing/

http://kimberlysnyder.net/blog/2012/09/22/9-foods-that-cause-inflammation-and-9-that-fight-it/

http://www.medicalnewstoday.com/articles/248423.php

http://www.webmd.com/arthritis/about-inflammation?page=2

http://www.ncbi.nlm.nih.gov/pubmedhealth/PMH0009852/

https://www.womentowomen.com/inflammation/causes-of-inflammation/

http://www.marksdailyapple.com/what-is-inflammation/#axzz3LHbGyhPY

http://www.nlm.nih.gov/medlineplus/ency/article/000438.htm

http://www.health.com/health/gallery/0,,20705881_2,00.html

http://www.britannica.com/EBchecked/topic/287677/inflammation/214909/Chronic-inflammation

http://lpi.oregonstate.edu/ss07/inflammation.html

http://courses.washington.edu/conj/inflammation/acuteinflam.htm

http://www.preservearticles.com/2012032028120/what-is-the-mechanism-of-acute-inflammation.html

www.ingramcontent.com/pod-product-compliance
Lightning Source LLC
Chambersburg PA
CBHW062008280526
45787CB00005B/2023